Health and Nutrition for Dogs and Cats

Health and Nutrition for Dogs and Cats

A Guide for Pet Parents

David G. Wellock

ROWMAN & LITTLEFIELD PUBLISHERS, INC.
Lanham • Boulder • New York • Toronto • Plymouth, UK

Published by Rowman & Littlefield Publishers, Inc.
A wholly owned subsidiary of The Rowman & Littlefield Publishing Group, Inc.
4501 Forbes Boulevard, Suite 200, Lanham, Maryland 20706
www.rowman.com

10 Thornbury Road, Plymouth PL6 7PP, United Kingdom

British Library Cataloguing in Publication Information Available

Library of Congress Cataloging-in-Publication Data Available

ISBN 978-1-4422-2086-7 (cloth : alk. paper)
ISBN 978-1-4422-2087-4 (electronic)

♾™ The paper used in this publication meets the minimum requirements of American National Standard for Information Sciences—Permanence of Paper for Printed Library Materials, ANSI/NISO Z39.48-1992.

Printed in the United States of America

Contents

Foreword

"Hi! I'm Jim Walker, President of Global Pet Foods," is how I've addressed radio listeners in Canada and the United States for almost a decade now, so it's an appropriate introduction here. Years ago, Global Pet Foods purchased a small pet food chain out of bankruptcy. The first franchisee we brought on board following the purchase was Dave Wellock, and I've had the pleasure of working with Dave ever since he started in the specialty pet food industry.

Dave's book, which I'm very pleased to introduce, chronicles his adventures along the way. It may seem odd to call the small retail shopkeeper learning process an adventure, but once you get into this book you'll understand what I mean. Dave started in the industry when, from a pet nutrition standpoint, it was really the "wild west." I love the detail of some of the ingredient lists that Dave comments on from the early days. Like me, I'm sure you'll get a few laughs with his funny little quips, such as the protein in some of these foods could quite possibly physically include his Auntie!

Dave's just that kind of guy who "calls 'em as he sees 'em"—and what a tale (mind the pun) it is. Over the years he's witnessed the wonderful evolution in pet foods as they've progressed toward more human grade, wholesome, and some might say "natural" ingredients; an evolution that has nutritionally benefited countless pets. Watch your phraseology though, as Dave will quickly point out that descriptive words like "natural" can be used to describe ingredients that few in their right minds would ever consider as having come from nature!

This book describes other deceptive practices, such as manufacturers splitting an ingredient into component parts to make it seem as if there's less of that ingredient in the diet. For example, back when Dave first started out, we carried a product that touted itself as the first fresh chicken diet in the marketplace. Unfortunately, fresh meat doesn't mix well with other dry components and won't form a kibble unless the water is reduced. When you add several forms of corn (all listed as separate items) you'll quickly come to realize that the diet really should have come to market as "Lots of Corn and a bit of Chicken Diet." While some manufacturers still get away with such deceptions, Dave's book will instruct concerned pet parents in avoiding these pitfalls.

Thanks to owner/operators like Dave, pet parents (or as Dave calls them, paropets) now have a fighting chance to feed their furry friends some of the best-prepared foods we've ever had the good fortune of selling! Dave's book is written in terms that will help you walk in his shoes as he goes from someone who's never been in the business to a true pet food professional. I have one final piece of advice. For any pet parent interested in identifying nutritious diets for their cat or dog—and learning how good nutrition influences overall pet health—read this book. It may be the only book on this subject you'll ever require.

I would like to thank Dave for his years of support and contribution to the education of not only his customers but also of fellow franchisees and friends like me who have had the good fortune to have him as a part of our team!

Jim Walker
President
Global Pet Foods

Acknowledgments

It would be impossible to write a book such as this without support and guidance from others. First, I wish to thank my wife, Penny, for the patience, perseverance, and encouragement that saw us through this project and innumerable other endeavors during the course of our lives together. Without her, many things would not have been possible. Credit also goes to my daughter, Heather. By skillfully taking on the management of our business, she provided me with the time needed to write this book.

My wonderful friend Jill Dennis, the Princess of Punctuation and Goddess of Grammar, reviewed every page for grammar/punctuation errors and readability, providing suggestions and remarks that kept me grounded and often generated a smile. She also makes killer peach jam. Jill, I promise to do all the cooking when next visiting.

Dr. Gary Pusillo, MS, PhD, PAS, ACAN diplomat, board-certified animal nutritionist, who was an acquaintance and is now a friend, took time from his very busy schedule to review much of the book for factuality, thus making this book better and more meaningful than it would have been otherwise. Remaining errors are mine alone. Every pet owner should hope Dr. Gary will write his own book . . . soon. Gary, IOU one fishing trip.

A thank you also goes to Jim Walker and the senior management team at Global Pet Foods. Your wisdom in allowing franchisees an opportunity to grow their own business, and importantly, enjoy personal grow within their own business, made this work possible in a very real sense. While change is always necessary, I hope you never lose that special vision that has made our expanding franchisee family so unique.

Having received several rejections from literary agents, it was exciting when Anne Devlin responded to my email with a request for additional information. Thank you, Anne, for seeing that which your peers missed, and for finding a publisher. A similar grateful thank you goes to senior editor Suzanne Staszik-Silva and the team of Elaine McGarraugh, Desiree Reid, and Kathryn Knigge at Rowman & Littlefield. They have been supportive, efficient, and professional at each step of the publishing process.

Finally, I owe a heartfelt thank you to my customers. Ours has been an interesting relationship. Sometimes my customers have been the teacher and I the student. Other times I have been the teacher, they the students. Without you, and your interest in the nutritional health of your furry family members, this book would never have happened.

Introduction

> I have been studying the traits and dispositions of the "lower animals" (so called) and contrasting them with the traits and dispositions of man. I find the result humiliating to me.
>
> —Mark Twain

Cats are aloof, arrogant, snoopy, persnickety, indifferent, fussy, uppity, intolerant, disdainful, superior, furtive, humorless, paranoid, egocentric, independent, determined, lazy, demanding, impatient, suspicious, and overly cautious.

Dogs are devious, treacherous, self-centered, tricky, greedy, dependent, impetuous, accepting, selfish, inconsiderate, sneaky, demanding, stubborn, underhanded, needy, scheming, thoughtless, and lacking any sense of decorum.

If you know people possessing only a few of the above attributes, you would cross a busy street at a dead run to avoid them. How is it then, in spite of possessing so many negative characteristics, we so dearly love our cats and dogs? The answer is simple. Our cats and dogs uncritically accept us for what and who we are by overlooking our many human flaws. In gratitude, we overlook theirs.

In 1998, having left an employer after working for them for many years, I decided, while driving home, that I was never going to work for someone else again. I was fed up with being underpaid and underappreciated. It was time to be my own boss, an exciting but intimidating prospect. It took almost four years of sweat, worry, sleepless nights, and sporadic bouts of fear to turn that entrepreneurial initiative into a good decision. Up until then, it was a bad decision.

As much of my working career involved sales and marketing, particularly in retail management, retail was my comfort zone. Thus, a suitable retail opportunity was my target as I commenced searching for self-employment. I eliminated things such as shoe stores, restaurants, and auto repair shops as such businesses fell well outside of my experience. Other opportunities eliminated me by requiring a financial investment exceeding my meager monetary resources.

I spent several weeks fruitlessly scanning newspapers, realty listings, and franchise publications before finally spotting a small advertisement offering a local pet supply store for sale. That interested me. I knew something about pets as, like most families, we had owned both dogs and cats. In fact, my shelter-rescued dog, Frisky, was lying on the floor a few feet from me as I contemplated the advertisement.

Frisky was, in a way, an ownership accident for my family. My wife and children had been pestering me for months to adopt a dog following the demise of our elderly cat, Busted (we named her Busted because, on the day after we adopted her as a small kitten, she knocked a china figurine off a table, shattering it on the tile floor). I was not in favor of a dog adoption just then, and I kept stalling. Finally, my wife put her foot down, stating that she and the children intended to drive to the local shelter to see if an appropriate four-footed canine family member was available. This, I was informed in no uncertain terms, was happening now. I was welcome to accompany them on this mission, an invitation that I declined.

My sole instruction as they headed out the door was "don't bring home a poodle." I'm unsure as to my motivation for those words. It was probably driven by testosterone, a macho self-image, or some other of my numerous male handicaps. Poodles weren't manly, or so I thought. I could defend my poodle-dismissive attitude, as we lived in a rural area at that time—big dog territory: large, self-sufficient, unkempt, fearless, manure-eating, surly, unrepentant, and disrespectful farm dogs surrounded us in all directions. Nobody posted "Beware of Dog" signs . . . that was a given.

I couldn't believe it! They brought home a poodle: black, miniature, a manly male with an abundance of macho attitude, as I would quickly learn. As soon as he crossed the threshold he assumed the role of Alpha Male, or perhaps even ALPHA MALE. I truly believe, when he passed away many years later, he still retained that assumption. What went wrong with my simple "no poodle" instruction? As I recall, here's how it happened.

> "That's the right size," said one. "Not too big and very friendly."
> "But it's a poodle. You know what Dad said about poodles."
> "Yeah, but it has its whole tail! With that tail, Dad will never guess it's a poodle."

Children and wives seem to have a global—perhaps universal—lack of respect for the intelligence of fathers. I'm boasting here, but I recognized the breed as soon as the dog came through the door. "What's this, a poodle . . . with a tail?"

I'd been poodled! By then it was too late for me to influence the decision. Enter Frisky, the undocked poodle, into our family. Now we were five, not counting the resident mice occupying the attic. The shelter folks claimed that Frisky was turned in by someone who witnessed him being tossed from the rear window of a slow-moving Cadillac. The more I got to know him, the more credible that story became, as there were a few times I wished I, too, owned a slow Caddy with which to take him for a one-way ride. Frisky never possessed anything like Cadillac class, but he certainly had a Mack truckload of character.

It's quite possible that among the five of us, Frisky had the highest IQ. For example, we left him alone in the house one day, along with a fresh loaf of Italian bread that was safely positioned on the dining room table. Arriving back home, we discovered Frisky had managed to get up on the table to visit the bread. Not a bite was missing from the loaf; being a genius, he knew it was worth his life. Instead, the crust was carefully punctured with a multitude of fang marks—horribly gummed over, but not one crumb missing. If he couldn't enjoy the bread, neither could we. We kept Frisky but threw out the bread. We still miss him in spite of his devious personality.

So yes, I was knowledgeable regarding cats and dogs. Further, thanks to the kids, we'd homed guppies, goldfish, hamsters, and a cat. I say "hamsters" because the healthy-looking lone hamster we brought home from the pet store turned out to be a female in an advanced state of pregnancy. One morning we discovered we'd gone from hamster to hamsters. I don't know if Blondie (mama hamster) was surprised, but my wife and I sure were. The kids, of course, were delighted with that turn of events. Thanks to Blondie, most of the neighborhood children ended up with a free pet hamster.

With such extensive, hands-on pet experience, a pet supply store seemed worth investigating. After some negotiation, I bought a down-but-not-totally-out pet supply business. The chain had gone bankrupt, and a competitor had purchased the assets. Most locations were quickly shut down, but they felt my location retained some potential, so it was put on the market. With a questionable future facing it, the price was right. The store had peaked at around $300,000 annual sales, but when I arrived on the scene it was down to less than half of that and still dropping . . . fast. Now I was an entrepreneur. Now I was self-employed. Now I had to find a way to turn around this failing business before I also became a failure.

In those years my new business, like most pet supply stores at the time, scraped by selling traditional national brands, most of which I subsequently learned were considered "grocery" brands—you could buy them anywhere. These diets were based on corn and enjoyed lots of corporate advertising but delivered little profit for a retailer. Additionally, there were a few food lines exclusive to small chains and independent pet retailers. These products were marginally more profitable than grocery brands and not as widely distributed, which helped stores like mine retain customers.

There were two things I learned rather quickly. First, being your own boss provides a great deal of satisfaction . . . but only if you're successful. When you're attempting to become successful, failure is always staring you in the face, and anxiety is a constant companion when you're living beneath The Cloud of Pending Doom. To this day I don't know how I managed to escape ulcers and a nervous breakdown. Second, my actual knowledge of pets before going into the business was nowhere close to what I thought I knew about pets. In hindsight, I was pet ignorant. I had a lot to learn.

I was about a year into the business, scraping by and making slow progress in increasing my sales, when a customer came in looking for a specific food I'd never heard of. I'd never heard of it because, at that time, high-quality diets were all but unknown in the market and totally unknown anywhere in my region. This customer, a dog breeder, kept returning, asking (nagging) me to bring this food line in for her. When I looked into it, I was shocked by the retail price they expected me to charge, as it was over $20.00 more per bag than anything else in the store. When I discussed it with a visiting sales rep, he told me I was crazy to even consider stocking such an expensive line. Who would spend that kind of money? Lots of people, as it turned out. I finally succumbed to my customer's pleas and brought the line into my store.

Thanks to that customer, the expensive line of dog food proved to be the first step in turning my business around. Sales picked up thanks to the word-of-mouth efforts of a grateful customer. Within months of that initial success I sourced a second line of quality food, then another. The store was on a roll, and it continues rolling along to this day. We've never looked back! We now see ourselves as a health food store for cats and dogs.

Today, almost fourteen years later, I'm still learning about cats and dogs and their nutrition and health issues. Much of the knowledge I have acquired over these years has come to me as a result of interaction with customers and their pets. My store became my school, and my customers and their pets my teachers. I thought it might be of benefit to share some of the things I've learned. Opinions on how and what to feed our pets abound. My opinions are anecdotal rather than scientific, based on my experiences in dealing with thousands of customers and their pets. Hopefully whatever passes for wisdom and insight on the pages of this book will benefit you, my fellow two-footers, in your dealings with those furry family members sharing your life.

Throughout the book you will meet Whiskers the cat and Spot the dog. They aren't my pets. They're your pets, or all pets. Early on in writing this book I became tired of using the words *cats* and *dogs* repeatedly, and decided Spot and Whiskers would introduce a little personality. I know, I know: Spot and Whiskers . . . how original is that? From time to time I mention Taffy. Taffy is my dog, now a fourteen-year-old cross between a Brittany spaniel and a Nova Scotia duck toller. Taffy, like all of my pets, was adopted from a local shelter. Taffy is a one-man woman; she sticks closer to me than does my shadow. In fact, when I had her with me in the store one day, an observant customer suggested I change her name to Velcro. I also mention Cinnamon, a springer spaniel who, like Frisky mentioned before, is now deceased. Cinnamon possessed a personality even a saint could envy if it wasn't for the fact that she would steal your donut in a heartbeat if you weren't careful (which shouldn't count against her as history shows that a good many saints weren't very saintly).

You will also discover I've created a new word—*paropet* (pronounced pare-o-pet)—which you will find in use throughout the pages of this book. I don't care to describe myself or others as "pet owners" because I don't see myself as "owning" Taffy any more than I own other members of my family. I am confident our dogs don't see themselves as being "owned," and if cats experience even a vague sense of ownership, it's them owning us. The term *pet parent* is too cumbersome for frequent use, so I reduced "parent of a pet" to *paropet*.

CHAPTER 1

The Rise of Pet Foods

The purity of a person's heart can be quickly measured by how they regard animals.

—Anonymous

There are many topics I'll be covering in the course this book, but as I've built my business on healthy, nutritious pet foods, it seems appropriate to start with food, a topic that continues to be near and dear to my heart. In the past decade, the introduction of unique new types of foods have created a tumultuous, confusing situation for consumers shopping in the pet food marketplace, a morass I will endeavor to guide you through in the following pages. But first, in order to have a suitable perspective on today's pet foods, a brief history lesson is in order.

Historically, dogs have been living with humans for at least fifteen thousand years and possibly more than twenty thousand years, not including that period when their gray wolf ancestors were motivated to lower their standards by associating with people. Dogs have the dubious honor of being our first domesticated companions. For humans, caves and other crude shelters were about as good as it got in terms of accommodation back when this relationship was developing. There were certainly no cities and no towns . . . not even small, permanent villages. We were hunter-gatherers. We fished, hunted animals large and small, and gathered grains, greens, nuts, insects, and fruits where we found them. We were constantly on the move from one foraging area to another. You might say our search for food motivated us to eventually populate the world. We ate anything and everything edible. When times were tough we even ate our dogs.

About twelve thousand years ago humans began moving from small hunter-gatherer groups to larger societies as a result of the development of agriculture in the Fertile Crescent, an area that covers much of today's Iraq and portions of neighboring countries from Turkey to Egypt. Our dogs moved right along with us, readily adapting to our changing environment . . . and our changing diet. Agriculture spread rapidly to Europe, Africa, and Asia as we learned how to domesticate grains such as wheat, oats, barley, and rice. The formation of small villages, larger cities, and eventually nations resulted from this initial agricultural success. This success was so important that wars were and are being fought over fertile farmlands and fickle water resources.

Having successfully domesticated dogs and grain, we humans were on a roll. Soon we were domesticating other animals such as chickens, cattle, horses, elephants, pigs, and sheep. Some of these animals were domesticated solely as food sources; others, such as horses, were predominantly a source of cheap labor. Dogs differed in that they were primarily companions to humans as fellow hunters and early warning systems, but they also provided labor, and sometimes, like horses, they became dinner. Throughout the centuries, our dogs have been eating what we've been eating, along with whatever tidbits they could forage on their own, such as a tasty rat, a crunchy apple, or a careless rabbit. As humans increasingly relied on a plant-based diet, we can assume their canine companions regularly ingested some of these foods as well.

Let me take this opportunity to clear up a popular misconception. A good many of my customers mistakenly believe their dogs are pure carnivores. This is true for cats but not quite so true for dogs. To the best of my knowledge all members of the canine family, while classed as carnivores, are actually more like omnivores where their stomachs are concerned . . . opportunistic omnivores in that canines can and do eat a wide variety of foodstuffs, even those living the wild life. That's why they have grinding molars in the rear of their jaws like bears and humans. I would agree that our dogs are meat-preferring omnivores, cheerfully ready to trot past the salad bar on their way to the roast pork, steak, or hamburgers. But if the meat has run out, some salad will do just fine, thank you.

Cats became domesticated at least ten thousand years ago, according to archeological evidence from Cyprus. As cats aren't native to that is land, we should assume domestication happened earlier, allowing cats to be imported from a mainland area, probably in the Fertile Crescent. One could argue that cats are self-domesticated, as those early felines were less interested in a relationship with us and more interested in the rodent populations enjoying the good life living off our stores of grain. I'm certain our ancient farming ancestors quickly recognized the benefits gained from allowing feral cats to keep populations of mice and rats in check, as too many rodents could quickly contaminate the fruits of months of tedious labor. Cats were welcome visitors who earned their keep by killing rodent pests. Eventually they moved into our homes and hearts. They caught their own meals, made few demands on us, and did their bathroom business somewhere off in the bushes. What's not to love? In many parts of the world, cats continue to perform this same valuable, centuries-old role. I recall reading a news report a few years ago regarding a plea to Vietnamese farmers by their government to stop eating their cats as the rural rodent population was growing out of control.

Cats, unlike dogs, are true carnivores. Actually, they're called *obligate carnivores*, as in "obligated to eat meat." Unlike dogs, cats have no grinding molars in their jaw, just sharp teeth designed to shred up a meat meal. Other obligate carnivores are animals such as crocodiles, raptors such as hawks, many fish species such as trout and sharks, all snakes, most bats, and even creatures that prey on insects, such as spiders. For cats, a bowl of corn meal is an insult to their stomachs.

So, after several millennia of cats self-feeding and dogs mooching our food, how did we get to today's commercial pet diets? It happened quickly . . . and recently. The first commercial pet food product, introduced around 1860, was a dog biscuit created by James Spratt, an American residing in England. His inspiration apparently resulted from witnessing dockyard dogs enjoying hardtack biscuits tossed to them by friendly sailors. Knowing what I do of the reputation of hardtack biscuits, I'm sure the sailors were as happy to get rid of them as the dogs were to receive them.

Thanks to Mr. Spratt, the idea was now out there; entrepreneurs commenced developing foods for pets. Commercial pet foods really came into their own following World War II. A booming postwar economy found an increasingly affluent society on the receiving end of a multitude of new products being introduced by large food companies, including new versions of pet foods. In most Western nations the population rapidly changed from a rural to an urban society housed in suburbs surrounding our expanding cities. We became commuters, forever hurrying to and fro, living a good portion of our lives on commuter trains or piloting our automobiles in the fast lane. As a part of these lifestyle changes, we increasingly became consumers of packaged foods, foods that allowed consumers to prepare meals in minutes rather than hours. Commercial pet foods benefited from this societal change. Dog biscuits, coarsely crunched up, became kibble. Canned meats, such as unwanted horsemeat, found a ready market as pet food. New products quickly evolved from those humble beginnings.

For the large food producers, creating pet food was more about profit and less about our pets. Unfortunately, too many of them still retain this attitude. Until the concept of commercial pet foods came along, tons of waste materials generated by companies making our human foods were simply dumped as garbage in landfills. The creation of pet foods meant that many food waste materials could now be put to a profitable use. What a clever idea! What's disturbing is that the practice is still in common use today, although it's no longer called waste; now we call them by-products, mill runs, and other names.

Food manufacturers now discovered a use for waste materials such as corn gluten meal and those animal parts unfit for the human food chain, such as intestines, skin, heads, feet, and even feathers. Additionally, some whole animals that couldn't be used at all in the human food chain were now useable in pet foods. These livestock animals are usually referred to as 4D animals. The term 4D stands for *dead*, *diseased*, *disabled*, and *dying*. For example, this would include a sick or dead cow found in a feedlot or a farmer's pasture, or a few dozen chickens that had suddenly died from an illness. Many small businesses still earn a living by collecting carcasses from farms and other sources and selling them to other businesses for rendering into pet-food ingredients.

That's bad enough. It gets even worse. In addition to collecting 4D animals for processing, these businesses also collected the carcasses of euthanized pets from veterinarians and animal shelters. Our beloved cats and dogs were themselves being rendered into pet food. I believe this disgusting practice is still allowed in some jurisdictions. It remains disturbing to me that our shelters and the veterinarian community are willing participants in such a despicable activity. While I can't recall it ever being mentioned, I don't know how such activity could be conducted for decades without the knowledge and approval of the primary organization in North America responsible for pet food regulations, the Association of American Feed Control Officials (AAFCO). Here's how AAFCO (www.aafco.org) describes itself:

> The Association of American Feed Control Officials (AAFCO) is a voluntary membership association of local, state and federal agencies charged by law to regulate the sale and distribution of animal feeds and animal drug remedies.
>
> Purpose and Function of AAFCO:
>
> Although AAFCO has no regulatory authority, the Association provides a forum for the membership and industry representation to achieve three main goals:
>
> - Ensure consumer protection
> - Safeguarding the health of animals and humans
> - Providing a level playing field of orderly commerce for the animal feed industry
>
> These goals are achieved by developing and implementing uniform and equitable laws, regulations, standards, definitions, and enforcement policies for regulating the manufacture, distribution, and sale of animal feeds— resulting in safe, effective, and useful feeds by promoting uniformity amongst member agencies.

While the majority of AAFCO voting members are state officials, there is also representation from Puerto Rico and Canada. Federal U.S. members include the Food and Drug Administration (FDA) and the Department of Agriculture. Nonvoting members include the National Grain and Feed Association, the Pet Food Institute, and the American Feed Industry Association. While all states are not members of AAFCO, most (if not all) nonmember states have adopted similar policies and guidelines.

Pet food manufacturers are supposed to follow AAFCO guidelines and policies for labeling and package statements and to use the Association's ingredient definitions and nutrition standards for pet foods, including feeding trials, which I will discuss later. The problem with guidelines and policies is that that's all they are—guidelines and policies, not enforceable laws. What's the downside for a company caught stepping out of line? Being a skeptic, I suspect penalties are nonexistent.

It is my opinion that the nutritional interests of our pets have not been well served by AAFCO. The extensive use of grain ingredients for our cats and dogs, ingredients that are better suited for ruminants like cattle and goats, or vegetation-first omnivores like pigs, has been approved by a controlling body whose foundation and primary interest is apparently more closely associated with the livestock and poultry industries. They approve ingredients, establish some standards, and dictate labeling requirements such as the guaranteed analysis (GA) shown on cans and bags of pet food (more on the GA later). However, one must wonder who benefits from AAFCO's approved ingredients, standards, and labels. I don't know about the benefits to the cows and chickens, but somehow I think our pets come up short on the benefit list. (Cattle are also losers here as I assume AAFCO regulations approved the feed ingredients that led to mad cow disease.)

In fairness, AAFCO doesn't make pet food. That's left to the whims of the pet food manufacturers who enjoy a generous list of raw ingredients from which to chose—some good, some bad. Manufacturers can opt to take the high road or the low road when it comes to decisions involving the quality of the ingredients they intend to use in their products. The question a paropet needs to ask is a simple one: does my pet or their shareholders come first in the company's thinking? For too many of us, we naively assume that the marketing promises regarding the quality of the diets offered are more than sufficient for maintaining good health for Whiskers and Spot. Have you ever read or watched an advertisement for pet foods stating they're using poor-quality ingredients that are unhealthy for your pet? Of course not! They're all using top-quality, healthy ingredients—or so they claim. Why not believe it? After all, we're not eating it. They make it very convenient to accept their statements at face value, an acceptance that may have negative consequences for your pet's nutrition. Other than as a reflection of cynicism, the words *truth* and *advertising* should never appear together in the same sentence.

Unfortunately, like much in marketing, the boastful health claims aren't necessarily true and may even be blatant lies. Paropets believe what the marketers tell us about our pet's diets because we believe what they tell us about our own diets. Excess sugar, salt, transfats, food colorings, chemical preservatives, and such are all good for us, or at least nutritionally acceptable, we are told. The marketing untruths and half-truths acquire creditability when rubber-stamped by our government agencies. As a culture, we've proven to be wonderfully gullible to the promoter's glib lies. The snake-oil salesmen and carnival pitchmen of old are alive and well . . . and working on Madison Avenue.

That was then! In the past fifteen years it has been interesting to observe that, as people have become more conscious of the benefits resulting from a healthier diet for themselves, they have also come to realize that the same basic health rules apply to their pets. We are increasingly suspicious of marketing claims directed at us for both our use and for that of our cats and dogs. As consumers, we are now more willing to challenge the deceitful claims pitched to us daily via print and electronic media. It's about time! We should be doing more of it.

As an example of marketing deception, our cats, as obligate carnivores, possess digestive systems designed for meat-rich diets. That grain-rich diets are freely marketed for cats has me convinced that a system for ensuring appropriate nutrition for Whiskers (and Spot) simply doesn't exist. While organizations such as AAFCO have a monitoring finger in the ingredient pie, I suspect nobody's watching the baker. That's our job. Today, if we're not informed consumers, we're uninformed dupes. Marketers can deceive us with impunity, and government support of consumers through labeling laws and policies is underwhelming, to say the least. I believe the Internet has done more to protect the consumer in the past decade than any government has done for us in the past century. The downside to the Internet is that much of what it provides is a babble of opinionated, misleading, or outright erroneous information, and both the positive facts and negative fictions remain in place forever, forcing us to become even more informed as consumers.

So let's commence the important process of assisting you in becoming an informed consumer where your pet's food is concerned. As we've touched on the use of grain in pet foods, and as grain has recently become a controversial pet food ingredient, we'll commence by exploring its role in pet diets.

GRAIN, GRAIN, AND MORE GRAIN

> You think dogs will not be in heaven? I tell you, they will be there long before any of us.
>
> —Robert Louis Stevenson

Today there continues to be a great deal of controversy over the use of grain in our pet foods, mostly relating to kibble, although canned foods are not exempt here. Fortunately, our pets have benefited from the controversy. While I'm not a fan of the overuse of grains such as corn and wheat in pet foods by profit-driven manufacturers, I don't see grain as being the monstrous evil some would have us believe. Somewhere, there has to be a sensible middle ground; the trick is to identify it.

As I asked previously, why are commercial grain-rich diets produced for obligate carnivores like our cats? The answer to that question can be provided with a single word . . . *profit*! What's good for our cats isn't really a part of the conversation. Recall, please, that for much of the past fifty years of the commercial pet food industry the purpose was to make a profit from what was formerly useless waste materials resulting from the production of human foods. In addition to these unused wastes providing no value to the company, the processed leftovers were probably a drain on profits, as the companies likely had to pay to dispose of them.

Grain is much cheaper than meat. Grain remnants from producing our foods, such as corn gluten meal and brewer's rice, are even cheaper than whole grain. The cheaper the ingredients, the greater the profit . . . simple enough! There's also a benefit for you, the buyer. Inexpensive grain and grain remnants used primarily as protein fillers in your pet's diet help keep your purchase price low, something we all care about. So guts and gizzards, feet and feathers—and grain—became the mainstay of the pet food industry for much of its existence: profitable for manufacturers, convenient and affordable for pet owners . . . and terrible for Spot and Whiskers.

The grain most commonly used in our pet foods is corn. In 2009, there were over eight hundred million metric tons of corn produced worldwide. Of that production, the United States alone accounted for over 40 percent, or about 333 million metric tons. That's a lot of bowls of corn flakes! (Actually, only a tiny percentage of all corn finds its way into the human diet.) It is the single largest grain crop in North America. Several years ago my son and I drove from Ontario, Canada, to southern California, where he would be working on a master's degree. My perspective of the American Midwest's interstate highways resembled a bobsled run. Bobsled runs are mounds of snow on either side of the icy track in front of you. All we could see in late August was the asphalt in front of us and a wall of green to the right or left as the highway cut a swath through endless miles of corn "as high as an elephant's eye." The corn seemed to go on forever. Occasionally, the visual tedium was broken when you topped a hill, allowing a momentary glimpse of farm buildings or trees off in the distance. Happily, corn doesn't grow on mountains; the Rockies finally appeared to break the monotonous "corny" scenery.

Because corn is plentiful, it is relatively inexpensive. Because it is inexpensive, it is widely used for poultry and livestock feed, and a multitude of other purposes, such as biofuel. Regrettably, our cats and dogs have all too often been lumped in with the poultry and livestock industry when it comes to feeding rules and regulations. Whiskers, Spot, and my dog Taffy may not be wolves and tigers, but they sure as hell aren't goats, either. Nonetheless, corn has, for much of the past fifty years, been a mainstay of the pet food industry. Other cereals such as wheat, rice, soybean, and sorghum are also commonly used in pet foods. I really don't mind a bit of grain in a pet food, not even cat food. What I really object to are pet diets that are predominately grain based, especially those incorporating low-quality grain by-products.

We will now go on a shopping trip to examine an assortment of dog and cat diets that will allow you to differentiate between the good, the bad, . . . and the ugly.

CHAPTER 2

Shopping for Your Pet's Food

> Don't accept your dog's admiration as conclusive evidence that
> you are wonderful.
>
> —Ann Landers

Good pet nutrition begins with knowing what's in the product. The single most important step required for you to become an informed consumer is to read and understand the information found on the packages and labels of pet foods. There is a great deal of information provided; some of it is valuable, some misleading, and some useless. In order to make an informed decision for feeding your cat or dog, you need to know which information is important and to understand the value of that information.

Preventing Spot or Whiskers from being fed like a cow or pig is actually a fairly easy process when you know what to look for. Your starting point for information should always be the ingredient list (IL) on your pet food package or label. Actually, reading ingredient lists is a good habit to get into when purchasing products for your own use. In the pet food industry, ingredient regulations are much the same as in our food industry. Why not? In many cases they share the same government regulators. The other option, of course, is to teach Whiskers and Spot to read, then they can do the shopping themselves. I wouldn't do this, though, as most of our pets are bossy enough as is; teach them to read and they may want to select what you and I eat for dinner tonight.

In my opinion the ingredient list provides some of the most relevant information presented to you on the package or label. For me, it's the first information I study when determining if the product is suitable for my pet, and equally important, suitable for my customers' cats and dogs. That being said, I'm the first to admit that there's a degree of trust involved in accepting the information provided here or anywhere else on the package. Trust is required because, as pointed out earlier, this information is the result of guidelines and policies rather than laws.

In North America, ingredients must be listed by weight in order of their contribution to the contents. If there's more meat by weight than rice, the meat will be listed first; if there's more corn by weight than meat, the corn will be listed first, and so on until you reach the end of the list. That's helpful up to a point. It doesn't prevent food producers from indulging in devious manipulations, apparently with the approval of our government regulators. (I'll explain this shortly.) It isn't enough to simply read the ingredient label; you also need to understand the information you're reading in order to determine if you are being manipulated.

The following is an ingredient list taken from a popular dog food product available in mass-market outlets: ground yellow corn, chicken by-product meal, corn gluten meal, whole wheat flour, animal fat preserved with mixed tocopherols (form of vitamin E), rice flour, beef, soy flour, sugar, propylene glycol, meat and bone meal, tricalcium phosphate, phosphoric acid, salt, water, animal digest, sorbic acid (a preservative), potassium chloride, dried carrots, dried peas, calcium propionate (a preservative), L-Lysine monohydrochloride, choline chloride, added color (Red 40, Yellow 5, Yellow 6, Blue 2), DL-Methionine, vitamin E supplement, zinc sulfate, ferrous sulfate, manganese sulfate, niacin, vitamin A supplement, calcium carbonate, copper sulfate, vitamin B12 supplement, calcium pantothenate, thiamine mononitrate, garlic oil, pyridoxine hydrochloride, riboflavin supplement, vitamin D3 supplement, menadione sodium bisulfite complex (source of vitamin K activity), calcium iodate, folic acid, biotin, sodium selenite.

Here's what I see in this ingredient list. The first and third ingredients are corn products, *ground yellow corn* and *corn gluten meal*. This inclusion of two similar ingredients is referred to as fractions in both the human and pet food industries. Here, they first provide ground whole corn, followed quickly with the less expensive corn gluten meal, the latter a processing leftover more appropriately relegated to a landfill site than a bag of pet food. While proponents supporting the use of corn gluten meal in our pet foods (pet food manufacturers using this ingredient appear to be the only ones supporting its use) can provide rational explanations for its inclusion, it's interesting to note that the ingredient is rarely, if ever, considered suitable for use in any human food products (at least I've never noticed it, and I am a food label reader). Frankly, if it isn't suitable for you or me, then it's not suitable for Whiskers or Spot, and possibly not even suitable for pigs or cows. Here is a simple description of corn gluten meal: a corn by-product created during the wet milling process used by the food-processing industry involved in producing corn starch and corn oils.

There is some justification here for consumers like you and me to assume that the use of grain fractions is a government-approved way for food manufacturers to deceive us. Look at some human products, such as cookies, and you'll see *sugar* high on the list, and further down other sweeteners such as *fructose*, *sucrose*, or *malt syrup* will be included in the ingredients. It's all sugar; they just don't want you to think about it that way. I suspect magicians have a name for this type of deception.

Another good example of ingredient splitting in a pet food might read: *lamb meal, white rice, brewer's rice, rice flour. . . .* In this example, in spite of using various forms of rice, it should be obvious that the total rice content by weight will likely be far greater than that of the lamb meal. When I see ingredient splitting on the list I instantly become suspicious as to what other deceptions this manufacturer is using to deceive me and to nutritionally cheat my pet.

Let's return to the above ingredient list. By the combined weight provided by its first and third position on the list, corn, in both of its forms, is clearly the dominant ingredient in this food. The fourth ingredient is another grain product, *wheat*, and the sixth is *rice flour*, with *soy flour* appearing even further along. Both flours represent highly refined products and are not as healthy as less-refined ingredients in the same way that white bread from highly refined flour is less nutritious than bread made from whole wheat flour. With four grain products represented in the first ten listed ingredients (versus a single meat product in the group), one might reasonably conclude that this is a corn-heavy, starch-rich, grain-based diet.

While not as high on the ingredient list as the grains, *soy flour* is present. There is justifiable concern among paropets regarding the inclusion of soy products in pet foods. Although soybean is an excellent source of plant protein, the jury is still out on its use in pet diets. Many believe soybean is difficult for pets to digest, and there is some evidence that it is likely a significant contributor to diet-induced pet allergies. Their fears may be valid, as there is concern with its use in human diets: The website for the Asthma and Allergy Foundation of America (aafa.org) states, "Soy (also called soya, soy bean, or glycine max), is among the most common foods that cause allergic reactions. Researchers are still not completely certain which component of soy causes the reactions, but so far 15 allergenic proteins have been found in soy."

As cats and dogs probably metabolize soy protein less efficiently than do humans, it should come as no surprise that it's even higher as a cause of allergies for pets than for humans (as shown in a later chapter on allergies). For a person or pet allergic to an ingredient, even a small amount of this ingredient could create a serious allergic reaction. That any pet food manufacturer would deliberately include a soy ingredient, in the face of obvious controversy, reflects a certain disdain for both our intelligence and the health of our pets. Regrettably, the disdain for our intelligence may be warranted, as the diet represented is popular with many paropets. Again, if you aren't an informed consumer, you could turn out to be an uninformed dupe. Similar allergy concerns exist for all forms of corn and wheat, all found in significant quantities in this diet. More on allergies in a later chapter!

Meat appears as the second ingredient in the form of *chicken by-product meal*. Meat by-products are all of the animal parts that can't be used in the processing of human foods. All of it! Chicken by-product meal can and often does include heads, feet, guts, feathers, and 4D birds. Some of this material may be partially decomposed. In fairness, nutritionally, organ meats are okay: I'm sure our cave-dwelling ancestors thought so. Heck, even some guts don't bother me as long as its content isn't excessive. In the wild, the guts and organs of a kill are a carnivore's equivalent of our fast food—quick to access, easy to eat. The remaining chicken parts belong in the nearest landfill, not in pet food.

In an effort to prevent any confusion here, allow me to explain the difference between chicken by-product meal and chicken meal as I've had many customers assume they are the same thing. Not so! As just mentioned, chicken by-product meal contains most of the undesirable parts of a chicken. On the other hand, chicken meal is basically chicken meat, and it is defined by AAFCO. Along with clean chicken flesh, it can contain some skin and bone. Feet, feathers, heads, and entrails will be missing. Both meals undergo a cooking process to separate fat from meat and to reduce moisture from about 70 percent to a level of approximately 10 percent, and then it's ground up into a meal, ready for sale to a pet food manufacturer. Chicken meal will have a protein content of about 65 percent compared to fresh chicken at about 18 percent, and a fat content of about 12 percent compared to 5 percent in fresh meat. The difference in values can be attributed to water content, which will be explained shortly. While chicken meal may not be perfect, it remains a vastly superior ingredient when compared to chicken by-product meal.

The fifth ingredient, *animal fat*, also bothers me. This is an unidentified fat that means it can come from any animal source, or even other sources such as restaurants or food processors. We, the consumers, have no idea as to what kinds of animals contributed to this ingredient, or what uses and processes the fat was subjected to prior to ending up as a pet food ingredient. I think we can all safely assume here that it was likely the cheapest animal fat source they could obtain at the time. Sadly, it's possibly a different concoction with each batch—inexpensive and unidentifiable, and deemed by some to be suitable for Whiskers and Spot. An additional problem with these mystery fat sources is the very real risk they've been preserved with chemical antioxidants such as BHA, which I'll discuss later in this chapter. If we're going to use an animal fat source, that's fine—I would like to see the source clearly identified as, for example, chicken fat.

This particular product is heavily advertised using pictures of nutritious vegetables, which appeals to your interest in providing a healthy food to your dog. The vegetable selection here is limited to carrots and peas, but you'll need to be a bit of a sleuth to locate them on the list above. Start at the beginning and work your way down the list. Keep working down . . . further . . . further. Don't give up! You're almost there, just a bit further. There they are, almost to the middle of the ingredient list. The position of these ingredients so far down the list is your first clue as to how insignificant the contribution of the peas and carrots is to your pet's nutrition if eating this food. Surprisingly, even some of the mineral and preservative supplements are higher on the list than are the vegetable ingredients. As the peas and carrots are included as "dried," they should retain their position on the IL. The seductive packaging suggests one thing—the truth presented by the ingredient list provides a different nutrition picture.

Why is *sugar* included in this diet? It isn't beneficial to your dog. Well, dogs share many things in common with people, which is probably a major reason why people and dogs get along so well. One commonality is enjoying foods that appeal to our sweet tooth. I'm of the opinion the sugar here is included purely as a flavor enhancer to improve palatability, as it will contribute nothing to Spot's nutrition and is likely detrimental to his overall health.

Another flavor enhancer found in this food is *animal digest*. What the heck is *animal digest*, some of you are wondering? Maybe you really don't want to know. Wikipedia bluntly describes animal digest as an ingredient commonly found in less-expensive pet foods. AAFCO defines it as material resulting from chemical and/or enzymatic hydrolysis of clean and undecomposed animal tissue. The animal tissues used shall be exclusive of hair, horns, teeth, hooves, and feathers, except in such trace amounts as might occur unavoidably in good factory practice and shall be suitable for animal feed.

What this means is that animal digest is really a broth made from parts of animals; animals that can be obtained from any source, with little or no control over quality or contamination as long as they aren't in a state of decomposition. Any poultry or mammalian meat sources can be used: 4D animals, goats, horses, dogs, cats, restaurant and supermarket refuse, and so on. If it wasn't illegal they could even toss Aunt Jill into the mix, just as long as they remove her bifocals first. Are you grossed out yet? I'm going to guess this explanation is everything you never wanted to know about animal digest. Its main purpose is as a flavor enhancer in pet and livestock foods. I have never seen animal digest used in what I consider to be a good-quality food. Do you still want to feed this food to Whiskers or Spot?

The *propylene glycol* also adds sweetness, but I suspect its primary role here is to provide a chewy, artificial meat texture to some food bits rather than the normal crunchy texture of kibble. Artificial meat texture! Hmmmm! Are we deceiving the pet or the pet owner? Frankly, the inclusion of a chemical like this in any pet food leaves me as cold as ice when I consider that it is being ingested day in, day out, for the pet's daily meals.

Warning: In addition to some pet foods, you may find propylene glycol in packages of treats, especially soft, moist pet treats and some dental treats. Even when buying pet treats, read the ingredient label.

So in this dog food formula, the sugar, animal digest, and likely some of the salt is included primarily as flavor enhancers. Why, then, are so many flavor enhancers required in this diet? It's not much of a mystery. As corn and overprocessed meat parts aren't likely your pet's first choice as a preferred meal, there has to be something in there to encourage him or her to eat it, thus the intentional addition of flavor enhancers. That these diets have often proven to be addictive benefits the manufacturer in that it becomes increasingly difficult for you to wean your pet off their food and onto competitor's brands. I can't see many dogs standing on their heads for this food without the addition of these ingredients whose insidious function is to increase the food's palatability while contributing little, if anything, to its nutritional health.

I refer to diets like this as "pizza diets"—with apologies to the pizza industry. We love pizza because of the huge flavor hit our taste buds receive when eating it; lots of fatty, tasty cheese, tomato sauce, and various flavorful toppings such as pepperoni, bacon, or pineapple. Don't forget the mushrooms, thanks. What's not to love? It certainly tastes great but, for your health, would you want to be eating pizza two or three times a day, every day, month after month for years? If you answer "yes," I have serious concerns regarding your longevity.

Another problem I have with this diet is the ingredient *meat and bone meal*. What's this stuff? Like the animal fat mentioned above, meat and bone meal is yet another mystery ingredient. It definitely falls under the indeterminate category of "stuff." It is pretty much exactly what you imagine; unidentified meat and bone ingredients all cooked down and rendered into a meal. Source unknown, quality unknown: a clamoring alarm bell for your suspicions! It's often added to pet foods when the initial meat ingredient (chicken by-product meal in the above ingredient list) is insufficient for the health of the animal. Here's a description of this unsavory substitute for an appropriate food ingredient provided by Ingredients101.com: "Meat and bone meal is the dried and rendered product from mammal tissues." Wikipedia notes the product is typically about 50 percent protein, 35 percent ash, 8 to 12 percent fat, and 4 to 7 percent moisture. It is primarily used in the formulation of animal feed to improve the amino acid profile of the feed. Feeding of MBM to cattle is thought to have been responsible for the spread of BSE (mad cow disease). In most parts of the world, MBM is no longer allowed in feed for ruminant animals. However, in some areas, including the United States, MBM is still used to feed monogastric animals. It is widely used in the United States as a low-cost meat in dog and cat food.

If potential mad cow disease isn't a sufficient turnoff, while not covered in the definition above, I'm guessing it's highly probable that meat and bone meal will also incorporate 4D animals in its composition, along with meat refuse from other sources such as meat-packing plants and other large-scale food processing facilities. While providing protein for Spot, in my opinion its inclusion here is due primarily to price. It's cheap! An additional concern here, as with similar mystery ingredients, is that chemical preservatives may be used to prevent the fat content of the MBM from becoming rancid until being used by a pet food manufacturer. And please remember, this disgusting ingredient is approved for pet food use by AAFCO.

Now, if all of that isn't bad enough, they're using four *food dyes* as ingredients. Count them yourself! I want you to think about that for a moment. Do you believe for a single second that the color of the food is important to your dog? Of course not! Not a single bit! Color is not a big item in Spot's life, especially where food is concerned. Dogs use their incredible noses for most of their eating decisions. If they like the smell, they'll eat it; if not, they won't. The assorted colors of the kibble in this particular food are for your benefit, even though you aren't likely eating the food! (While some pet foods will enhance your overall diet, this isn't one of them.) The red bits look meaty, the green ones look like healthy vegetables. Dig in! Enjoy! Why should your dog have all of the good stuff? The dyes are included here so that the food appears healthy and nutritionally attractive to you, providing you with the false belief that you're being a good pet parent by conscientiously feeding a healthy food.

I guess we really can't blame these pet food manufacturers for such deceptions as similar deceits are used by those producing our packaged human foods (check out children's cereals on your grocer's shelves) and are always government approved. Still, these dyes are of no benefit to your pet (or children) and shouldn't be there.

That's the game then! In my opinion this is a heavily grain-based dog food diet masquerading as a healthy meal for your favorite four-footed companion. There's too much grain, the combined weight of which easily outweighs the meat ingredients. And the meat is of poor quality, including mystery meat sources, some of which may have 4D origins and chemical preservatives (discussed shortly). Sugar, by-product protein fillers, chemicals, suspicious flavor enhancers, an undesirable soy ingredient, mystery fats, and unneeded dyes round out the list of ingredients I find objectionable. It's enough to make a hungry dog weep. Finally, the vegetables they so proudly display on the package appear unimpressively far down on the actual ingredient list, making them almost valueless as a nutrition source. In short, I wouldn't feed this food to any living creature unless it was absolutely starving and nothing better was close at hand. And I would apologize while feeding it.

I have avoided discussing the various vitamin and mineral supplements included in the above ingredient list as, for the most part, they are presumably included out of necessity due to their loss or reduction in the process required to produce the food. While there is some variation in the vitamin/mineral cocktail added to foods by the various pet food manufacturers, they are all similar and serve a similar need to ensure basic (minimal) standards for nutritional health are being met. We do much the same when we add vitamin and mineral supplements to many human foods found on our supermarket shelves.

Traditionally, the above diet, and for decades most other pet food diets then (and still) marketed, were all similar. Some are even worse than that just reviewed. For example, only a few short years ago there was a forty-pound bag of dog food sold by a large retail chain that cost less than an equivalent-sized bag of pigeon feed. Lucky pigeons, unlucky dogs! The dubious quality of the ingredients and the predominant reliance on cheap grains as the backbone of the foods leave much to be desired. Such ingredients, along with the chemical antioxidant preservatives commonly in use in the pet food industry in those years, notably ethoxyquin and the butylated twins (see definitions below), could be considered as actually being toxic for our pets. The good news is that there are now many better-quality diets available for our pets. The bad news is that poor quality diets are still prevalent in the marketplace . . . and clearly dominate the advertising.

While difficult to find anything nice to say about the diet presented above, at least this producer isn't using any of the chemicals for fat preservation still approved for use in pet foods. These are

- **ethoxyquin:** This is a quinoline-based antioxidant that is commonly used as a preservative in pet foods to prevent the rancidification of fats. It also has a role as a pesticide.
- **BHA and BHT:** Butylated hydroxyanisole (BHA) and the related compound butylated hydroxytoluene (BHT) are phenolic compounds that are often added to foods to preserve fats.

It is rare to see any of the above three chemical preservatives on pet food labels today. We call that progress! These chemicals are still in use, though, including in human products, although I understand that the level of chemical allowed in our foods was always much, much lower than that allowed for our pets. You may also find them used in low-quality soft, chewy pet treats. There remains justifiable suspicion that these chemicals can still be found at unacceptable levels as antioxidant preservatives in preprocessed pet food ingredients such as meat and bone meal, animal digest, and animal fat. Any mystery ingredients included in your pet's food should give you cause for concern regarding both the ingredient's quality and potential chemical content. The only way for concerned paropets to prevent their pets from ingesting such chemicals is to not purchase products with inexpensive or unidentifiable meat and fat ingredients. While that step may not be foolproof, it certainly reduces the risk to Spot and Whiskers.

Concerned pet parents had serious health issues related to the use of ethoxyquin, BHA, and BHT. These chemical preservatives, at the high levels allowed for use in pet foods, were suspected of being carcinogenic and especially detrimental to the health of pregnant pets and their offspring. Once the hue and cry was raised by paropets over the use of ethoxyquin, BHA, and BHT as preservatives, pet food manufacturers quickly stepped up their game by finding substitutes. The antioxidant preservative most commonly used to prevent fat going rancid in pet foods today is *mixed tocopherols*. You will find it associated with the chicken fat in both the above and following formulas. Customers have frequently asked for an explanation of mixed tocopherols. Basically, it is vitamin E. Vitamin E comes in eight different forms. Rather than reading it as "mixed tocopherols," look at it as though it states "mixed vitamin E." You will frequently see it used in conjunction with other natural preservatives such as extracts of rosemary or sage, vitamin C, and ascorbyl palmitate.

As for the diet described above, I personally would not, as in NOT, feed it to my dog. Frankly, I might feed it to the neighborhood crows, but only if I was in a crow-hating frame of mind on any given day.

Congratulations! You're on your way to becoming an informed pet food consumer. There are a few more steps to take, though. Now that we've taken a hard look at what I consider an inappropriate canine diet, let's examine a product I would feed to Taffy: chicken, brown rice, lamb meal, oatmeal, barley, potatoes, carrots, chicken fat (preserved with natural mixed tocopherols), duck meal, tomato pomace, natural flavor, canola oil, brewer's yeast, duck, salmon meal, sodium chloride, potassium chloride, salmon oil, whole ground flaxseed, choline chloride, taurine, natural mixed tocopherols, spinach, parsley flakes, cranberries, l-lysine, l-carnitine, yucca schidigera extract, dried kelp, vitamin E supplement, iron proteinate, zinc proteinate, copper proteinate, ferrous sulfate, zinc sulfate, copper sulfate, potassium iodide, thiamine mononitrate (vitamin B1), manganese proteinate, manganous oxide, ascorbic acid, vitamin A supplement, biotin, niacin, calcium pantothenate, manganese sulfate, sodium selenite, pyridoxine hydrochloride (vitamin B6), vitamin B12 supplement, riboflavin (vitamin B2), vitamin D3 supplement, folic acid.

Let's discuss the meats first. This diet contains five meat ingredients, all of them identifiable: no mystery meats are found in this ingredient list. The first ingredient, *chicken*, will be fresh chicken that contains no 4D animals or undesirable parts of the chicken such as feathers, bones, heads, entrails, and feet. Of the first ten ingredients, three of them, *chicken*, *lamb meal*, and *duck meal*, are better-quality meat sources than if containing inferior meat by-products, thus enhancing the recipient's nutrition.

A brief discussion is required here regarding the first ingredient, chicken. Any fresh meat is a heavy ingredient in that fresh meat is predominantly water, as per the USDA website (usda.gov) information below:

WATER CONTENT OF MEAT AND POULTRY
Raw cooked chicken fryer, whole, 66 percent
White meat chicken, with skin, 69 percent
Dark meat chicken, with skin, 66 percent
Ground beef, 85 percent lean, 64 percent
Ground beef, 73 percent lean, 56 percent
Beef, eye of round, 73 percent
Beef, whole brisket, 71 percent
The balance of that fresh meat is made up of protein, fats, and minerals.

Why am I bothering you with this information? Well, some manufacturers use the ingredient "fresh meat" as a marketing gimmick. "Fresh Chicken Is Our First Ingredient" is the type of phraseology you might find prominently displayed in their advertisements and blatantly presented on their bags of food. Its purpose is to favorably impress you, but the good impression may well mask a nasty deception.

Here's the problem. The fresh chicken, at almost 70 percent water going into the recipe mixture, is very heavy compared to the other ingredients that, excepting for the fat and vegetables here, are dry, and as a result, by weight they will legally qualify as the first ingredient on the ingredient list. However, the average moisture content of most dry pet foods is usually about 10 percent. So when that fresh meat in the first ingredient is cooked down to its final kibble form, it no longer possesses the water-rich weight advantage it enjoyed in its uncooked form: it will no longer be the first ingredient when going into your pet. The fresh meat is now about one-fourth of its former weight; therefore one pound (sixteen ounces) of the fresh meat that qualified for first place on the ingredient list now weighs in, at best, at about four ounces . . . a weight loss of about 75 percent. As we don't know how much fresh meat was initially provided, we can't calculate its cooked position on their ingredient list, but we should assume it has dropped several positions. That's why it's important to check for the inclusion of additional meat sources and the quality of them.

As pointed out, except for the potatoes, carrots, and fats, most of the other ingredients here are dry. Therefore, it doesn't take much fresh meat to qualify as the first ingredient. In order to ensure there are sufficient meat protein sources in the diet to satisfy the pet's health requirements, you will usually discover—when fresh meats are used— additional sources of meat protein. That's fine as long as those meats are also of good quality. You don't want to find meat by-products or, worse, mystery meat and bone meal as used in the prior diet. For those manufacturers using *fresh meat* purely as a marketing gimmick, you will usually discover that any additional meat ingredients are of poor quality. Fortunately, in this diet, all of the additional meat sources are of an acceptable quality when compared with the prior diet; we are not being subjected to a marketing deception.

Now let's take a look at some of the other items I like in this recipe. The second ingredient, *brown rice*, is the best form of rice for your dog's nutritional health. It is the whole grain including the rice bran, preferable to white rice and far superior to a rice by-product often used in lower-quality pet foods, brewer's (or brewers) rice.

Brewer's rice is the small, milled fragments of rice kernels that have been separated from the larger kernels of milled rice. Brewer's rice is a processed rice product that is missing many of the nutrients contained in whole ground rice and brown rice, thus reducing the quality. Brewer's rice is sold for pet food and dairy feed exclusively.

Oatmeal is a beneficial ingredient here. In addition to being a source of B vitamins, soluble fiber, and other nutrients, I have never found it to contribute to allergies in dogs. *Barley* contains eight essential amino acids as well as other nutritional benefits. As barley is one of the grains first cultivated by humans in the Fertile Crescent, it has probably been a part of many canine diets for centuries. Like oatmeal, I have never found barley to contribute to canine allergies.

While the *potatoes* and *carrots* are relatively high on this ingredient list, they are even more water rich than the chicken. (Potatoes are approximately 85 percent water.) Like the fresh chicken, once these vegetables are cooked down to the kibble's approximately 10 percent moisture content, they will be much further down on the list of ingredients going into the dog than many of the dry ingredients. Their inclusion in this food may be more for your benefit than that of your pet, as their nutrition contribution may be minimal at best. I'd be happier if there was no potato content at all.

The *salmon oil* and *flaxseed* are excellent sources of omega-3 fatty acids. That they use ground whole flaxseed here ensures that nutritional benefits from the seeds are presented in a form that can be maximized by the dog's digestive system. The *canola oil* also provides some omega-3. It's worth noting here that the plant and fish sources of omega-3 vary somewhat in their nutritional makeup, so inclusion of both sources here is beneficial for your pet.

The *cranberries* provide two benefits. They are a wonderful source of antioxidants and may serve to support the urinary tract.

While this diet isn't perfect, I would definitely feed it to my dog. In fact, Taffy has enjoyed this particular food on many occasions. When Taffy was thirteen years old her vet described her as "a poster child for good nutrition." I realize that, at the height of the current grain-free diet fad, this food will not meet with the approval of many. Sorry, I'm unconcerned, as the grains provided here do not dominate the ingredients. It's a fine diet, one that most pets would thrive on.

We've now examined a poor-quality traditional dog food and a good-quality contemporary dog food (a similar examination of cat diets would produce similar results). What's the difference? In a nutshell, the difference comes down to the ingredients used to make the food. The quality of the meat sources, quantity and quality of grain sources, along with the absence or inclusion of other healthy ingredients are the features you, the paropet, should be on the lookout for, as these are the elements that separate good diets from bad.

The word *quality*, be it good or poor quality, is subject to interpretation by each reader. When discussing pet foods, my definition of quality includes the following:

- If grains are used, they should be whole grains; no heavily refined grains or grain by-products.
- If fruits and vegetables are used, they should be table grade and biologically appropriate for Whiskers or Spot.
- Meats should be identifiable by animal source, no by-products or mystery meats.
- Fats should be identified by source; no generic sources, please.
- Dyes, sweeteners, questionable chemicals, and flavor enhancers are not used (especially flavor enhancers made from waste protein material).
- Vitamin E (mixed tocopherols) is the main preservative, rather than chemicals such as ethoxyquin.

I would also caution readers that price is not a useful guideline for quality. It is reasonable to assume that a product containing good meats and other whole foods will cost significantly more than one relying heavily on inexpensive grains such as corn and wheat and cheap protein fillers such as corn gluten meal or brewer's rice, along with questionable (mystery) meat ingredients. That's the way it should work. Unfortunately, there is no law preventing a manufacturer of poor-quality pet diets from charging a price comparable to that charged for a superior diet. Further, they can advertise a poor-quality diet as being a healthy, high-quality diet. Trust me; it's done every day. In today's world, the price tag for a national advertising campaign can run into the millions of dollars. Great packaging and even greater advertising may well be masking an inferior product. The only person who can protect you from being financially shortchanged and your pet from being nutritionally ripped off is you. The old saying "knowledge is power" has never been more true.

Now we'll examine some additional contemporary diets awaiting you at your pet's grocery store.

GRAIN-FREE DIETS

In the past few years the trending in cat and dog diets has been toward grain-free products. Due to their growing popularity, I would be remiss in my duty to make an informed consumer of you if I failed to cover a grain-free diet. As we've reviewed two canine diets, let's take a look at a feline food: chicken meal, russet potatoes, boneless chicken, boneless walleye, whitefish meal,* peas, chicken fat (naturally preserved with vitamin E), sun-cured alfalfa, chicken liver, boneless Lake Whitefish, whole eggs, salmon oil, sweet potato, pumpkin, spinach, turnip greens, tomatoes, carrots, apples, organic kelp, cranberries, blueberries, juniper berries, black currants, chicory root, licorice root, angelica root, fenugreek, marigold flowers, sweet fennel, peppermint leaf, chamomile flowers, lavender flowers, summer savory, rosemary, vitamin A, vitamin D3, vitamin E, niacin, zinc proteinate, thiamine, mononitrate, riboflavin, vitamin B5, iron proteinate, vitamin B6, manganese proteinate, copper proteinate, folic acid, biotin, vitamin B12, selenium, dried Lactobacillus acidophilus fermentation product, dried Enterococcus faecium fermentation product. *Whitefish meal contains wild-caught flounder, halibut, and cod.

Gee! I don't eat this well every day. You will note that while some fruits and vegetables are included in this recipe, no grains are present.

The first ingredient here is *chicken meal*. That's fine, as it should be free of meat by-products. The meal is already a dried product, so, unlike fresh chicken meat, it will not shrink much, if at all, on the ingredient list after the cooking process is complete. We can retain some confidence that our cat will be getting more chicken than anything else. For an obligate carnivore, this is very important.

The third and fourth ingredients are fresh chicken presented as *boneless chicken* and fresh fish in the form of *boneless walleye*; both are great, but they will cook down, as previously mentioned for any fresh meat source. (Canadian readers note that walleye is commonly called pickerel in most of Canada.) The fifth ingredient is a good-quality *whitefish meal* that, like the chicken meal, will retain its position on the list and in fact may move up the ingredient ladder as the fresh ingredients, when cooked, move down. It's also important to note here that the source of this fish meal is identified with the asterisk as wild-caught flounder, halibut, and cod; no guessing required. Further along, there is some fresh *chicken liver*, *Lake Whitefish*, and *whole eggs* to provide an overall terrific meat protein meal for a cat. All are quality foods with no mystery meat sources. Note that when it states "whole eggs" it can mean the whole egg . . . shell and all. There's nothing wrong with that, as the shell is a natural source of calcium.

The second ingredient is *russet potato*. Even more than fresh meat, potato is a water-rich product, with a water content of almost 85 percent. Once cooked down to the kibble's lower moisture content, the potatoes here will be well down the ingredient list when heading down the cat's throat. Still, I remain a skeptic when it comes to feeding potatoes to an obligate carnivore, particularly when it's a high-glycemic ingredient. What's *alfalfa* doing on this list? Actually, alfalfa is loaded with a multitude of minerals and trace elements, but its benefit for a carnivore, like the *marigold flowers* and other herbal and fruit ingredients, is questionable. While some of these ingredients may provide a nutrition benefit for a cat, I suspect their main role is to sexy up the diet to impress the paropet.

The *salmon oil*, again, is a great source of omega-3 fatty acid, vital for overall health and great for the cat's skin and coat. While a healthy coat doesn't prevent hairball formation, it certainly helps to reduce the incidence of hairballs, which are an unpleasant issue for many cats and pet parents. If you step on an upchucked hairball while stumbling around the house in the early morning you'll quickly understand what I'm talking about.

Lactobacillus acidophilus and *Enterococcus faecium* are digestion-friendly bacteria. All mammals have them; all mammals need them for good digestive health.

Would I feed this to my cat (if I had a cat)? Yes! Definitely! All of the ingredients are of good quality. Ample meat protein sources suitable for a carnivore are provided, combined with a suitable selection of other healthy whole foods. It might be a challenge moving your cat from a pizza-type diet to something as nutritious as this, but if your cat will eat it, I am confident you'll have a healthier pet.

Grain-free diets were developed to compete with the raw diet trend that appeared several years ago. It's interesting to note that, for years, pet food retailers like me, along with paropets, were asking manufacturers why more meat content wasn't included in their dog and cat foods. The standard industry response was that too much meat gummed up the extrusion equipment. It's ironic, then, when Natura Pet introduced Evo, the first grain-free cat and dog food kibble line, their competitors quickly followed suit by introducing their own grain-free products. I don't believe for one second that the competition could formulate a new food and retool their production equipment literally overnight. Call me a cynic, but I think it's more likely that we were deceived all along. Lower meat content means lower costs and greater profits for the manufacturers. It also helped keep the costs down for you, the buyer. Until Evo arrived on store shelves, manufacturers had failed to realize that many consumers wanted improved protein content in their pet's food and were prepared to pay for it. Their demands brought new meaning to "show me the beef!"

RAW DIETS

The introduction and rapid rise of raw pet food diets was an interesting phenomenon within the pet food industry. While raw food for dogs was proposed in the early 1930s, it didn't really find an interested community of any size until Ian Billinghurst, an Australian veterinarian, published *Give Your Dog a Bone* in 1993. They say timing is everything. Dr. Billinghurst's book appeared on the scene as a growing number of people were becoming increasingly concerned with the quality of their own diets. The sudden interest and demand for raw diets was a game changer for, up to then, a somewhat staid manufacturing community. Personally, I have to confess I was slow off the mark in introducing raw diets as a part of my store's product lineup. Mark it down to my skeptical nature. Initially, when raw diets first commenced appearing, most raw feeders early into the program were making their own pet diets at home as commercial production had not yet commenced. This created a great deal of concern because veterinarians were seeing more and more pets showing up in their clinics with serious, food-related illnesses.

Next, an increasing number of small businesses sprang up to make raw pet food diets. Many of these businesses were Mom and Pop operations, making raw pet foods out of their own homes using recipes created by themselves or sourced from the Internet. All too often, these producers had a great deal of enthusiasm but little or no prior commercial food preparation experience. They sometimes used unsuitable equipment when preparing these foods and had limited pet diet and nutrition knowledge, resulting in yet more sick pets showing up at vet clinics. As an example, one local raw pet food producer is reported to have been using a small, secondhand cement mixer in his garage to blend his ingredients!

Sadly, I have had three customers who lost dogs to raw diets. Salmonella and other dangerous bacterial food contaminants are as deadly to our pets as they are to us if the contamination level is high enough. In fairness, though, I will point out that in all three cases the dogs were on homemade raw diets versus quality commercial foods.

As well as bacterial contamination, intestinal parasites can be sourced from raw foods, including raw meats. While less probable from professional, commercially prepared meals, homemade raw diets may harbor unwelcome intestinal intruders if the meat source—designed to be cooked—is served uncooked. So, from my point of view, raw diets were off to a bad start. I didn't introduce raw diets for sale in my store until larger, professional manufacturers entered the field. Let's look at an appropriate, professionally formulated raw diet, suitable for both cats and dogs: lamb, lamb liver, raw ground lamb bone, lamb heart, lamb kidney, apples, carrots, butternut squash, ground flaxseeds, montmorillonite clay, chicken eggs, broccoli, lettuce, spinach, dried kelp, apple cider vinegar, parsley, honey, salmon oil, olive oil, blueberries, alfalfa sprouts, persimmons, duck eggs, pheasant eggs, quail eggs, inulin, rosemary, sage, clove.

As this is a frozen raw diet, the fresh meats will not be reduced in weight by cooking as they would in a kibble food; in fact, all ingredients will retain their positions on the ingredient list. There are no preservatives, like the mixed tocopherols noted earlier, as the freezing is the preservative. These diets are complete and are usually presented from the package in serving-sized portions for convenient feeding. As with any raw meat product, defrosting slowly in the refrigerator rather than on a kitchen countertop is always the safest method. Take out the breakfast meal the evening before and let it defrost in your fridge overnight. Take out the evening meal in the morning and let it defrost in your fridge all day.

Tip: Cats and dogs should not be fed defrosted or partially defrosted food that is cold. Place it in your microwave for a few seconds to bring it up to room temperature.

Most of the ingredients in this diet should be self-explanatory. Both muscle meat and selected organ meats (*heart* and *kidney*) are included.

The ground bone will provide an appropriate, natural source of calcium. Most of the ingredients preceding the clay will enhance the overall nutritional profile of the meal, including providing important antioxidants. The *montmorillonite clay* is a colloidal silicate with an extremely fine texture and contains over fifty ultratrace minerals. (It has also been found to bind aflatoxins; not an issue as grains are absent from the recipe.) Most of the ingredients following the clay will be present in insignificant amounts, thus they will not make much in the way of a nutrition contribution to your pet. Again, I suspect their role here is to dress up the diet to impress the purchaser.

Warning: An important point to remember when feeding raw meat is that it must be handled with EXTREME care. A failure to take proper precautions may result in serious food poisoning for your pet . . . and your family, should any toxins manage to transfer to your food supply. This is one of the reasons I caution pet owners with small children in the home to rethink feeding raw diets to pets (at least until the children are old enough to avoid the danger). Even something as simple as a small child playing for a few seconds with an empty pet food dish that held raw meat can create a serious health problem. Wash your hands thoroughly after contact with the raw food and carefully wash out the pet's food dish IMMEDIATELY after use. Remove and discard uneaten food within thirty minutes of serving (do not retain for a future meal).

It is the danger of handling and feeding raw meat, as well as the inconvenience, that has turned many off of raw diets and led directly to the creation and success of alternative foods, which we will discuss shortly.

Still, in spite of the inconvenience and danger, raw feeders are a dedicated group of aficionados: some would even qualify as zealots. That's a creditability problem for me. It commences with their belief that our dogs are only fifteen minutes away from being wolves, rather than fifteen thousand years, and, as such, will do best on a heavy raw meat and raw fat diet with a small bit of other foodstuffs tossed in for good measure. Their goal is the attempt to reestablish the dog's ancestral diet. That's the part I don't get. Remember, dogs have been eating what we've been eating for at least fifteen thousand years. Our human digestive system has altered to adapt to our dietary changes over the millennia. Our distant human ancestors started out as foragers and scavengers, later increasing their protein intake as they became efficient hunters, and finally moving to the convenience of a grain-based diet about twelve thousand years ago.

Is there any reason to think that our dogs haven't adapted? Of course they have. Thai dingo dogs (the ancestors of Australia's dingoes), for example, live nicely on a diet that's predominantly rice and bananas, and they probably consider themselves fortunate if even 20 percent of their food is meat. Also, an article I read years ago stated that some gray wolf populations in Europe and the Middle East have thrived for generation after healthy generation dining off food scraps in their local town dump, an easier way of making a living than killing chickens and sheep, as such activities would soon have the local two-footers collecting wolf pelts. Further, while watching a documentary on television a few years ago covering the lives of a pack of wild African jackals, the show noted, after people analyzed the jackals' scat over a period of time, that those canines enjoyed a diet in which meat ranged from 100 percent, when they could infrequently scavenge a lion kill, to 0 percent when they were forced to live off grasses and sedges. Much of the time, their diet was very light on animal protein, with the meat protein they could acquire coming from the occasional unwary small animal they killed, and insects. This convinces me that dogs are dogs, wolves are wolves, humans are humans, and bonobos are bonobos. Let's avoid deceiving ourselves into believing otherwise.

Look at it this way. In the fifteen thousand years since we first teamed up with our dogs, there have been approximately 375 human generations, if you allow an average lifespan of forty years over the centuries. In the same time period, allowing for an average lifespan of six years for dogs, there would be approximately 2,500 canine generations. That's about seven dog generations for each one of ours. When you come right down to it, our dogs have had a better opportunity to adjust to our diets than have we. I have no personal need to eat like a wild chimpanzee, and don't believe my dog will have a better life eating like a wild wolf, even one with the luxury of a town dump available.

This debate has been predominantly about dogs. For the most part, cats manage to escape the ancestral diet issue. As in most things, cats remain above the fray, comfortable in their superior knowledge of who they are and from whence they came. They are obligate carnivores— meat eaters. I've always suspected cats are aliens from a distant solar system. For them, we're cheap entertainment.

The problem is that these raw-feeding zealots loudly promote raw diets as the end all in feeding your cat or dog. The benefits claimed include cleaner teeth, better digestion, better stools, no allergies, fewer diseases, and better weight. Of the above claims, the only one I can lend credence to is that of obesity. Raw diets (at least those with high protein) will likely benefit most overweight pets needing to drop a few pounds. But then, so will other high-protein diets such as grain-free diets and baked foods.

A quick comment is required here regarding clean teeth, a favorite topic of raw feeders (their other favorite topic is poop). Neither of the two dogs that have shared my life since I purchased my store has ever needed to have their teeth cleaned by their veterinarian. Cinnamon, a springer spaniel, died at twelve years from a tumor. Taffy, who you've already met, is a fourteen-year-old who still sees herself as a puppy. Of course, both have been eating high-quality, low-grain and grain-free diets since they joined my family, at four and five years, respectively. I believe starchy, grain-rich diets are a cause of dental problems in cats and dogs. I can't prove it, but you can't convince me otherwise. Many starches are sticky and can adhere to teeth. (Dental issues are covered in a later chapter.)

Additionally, contrary to the raw feeder's beliefs, not all cats and dogs like their food raw—at least not when first introduced to it if they've been eating cooked foods. Your alternative, if you wish to avoid a kibble-style diet, is to lightly cook the raw food. You can do this in the microwave (fastest), oven, or frying pan. It won't be a true raw diet, but if you gently cook it, the food will provide nearly all of the benefits assumed to be associated with raw. Further, if you cook it less and less over a period of a week or two, you can probably wean your pet onto a purely raw, uncooked food. All you need is patience.

Finally, if ancestral diets are so beneficial, why aren't the supporters of such diets also feeding themselves an ancestral diet? If dogs should be eating like wolves, then it makes sense that these dog owners should be eating like hunter-gatherers by living on nuts, berries, roots, bugs, and some scavenged, fly-infested meat that's been in the sun too long. Nope! They want their pizza and ice cream, thank you!

As there has been little in the way of clinical studies to support or disprove the claims associated with feeding a raw diet to cats and dogs, I'm certain the debate will continue well into the future.

BAKED DIETS

Baked foods are the coming new players for the pet food industry. They are much like raw diets in formation and ingredient selection. Instead of being presented in an uncooked form, they are baked. Like raw diets, baked foods are sold in a frozen state. Defrosted, the product looks— and often smells—just like your favorite meat loaf, which is pretty much what it is. If someone served it up to you with mashed potatoes on one side, and peas and carrots on the other side, and if you didn't know better, you'd eat it with gusto . . . and a bit of ketchup.

Baked diets have an important advantage over raw diets in that the cooking process destroys any harmful bacteria and parasites associated with serious illnesses. Other advantages over raw worth noting are that these diets, not being contaminant-dangerous to pets and small children, are safer to handle and more convenient to serve. By incorporating minimally processed whole foods, quickly frozen to retain freshness and palatability, baked diets are highly beneficial for our pets' nutritional health. While the baking process may degrade some of the nutritional benefits when compared to raw, the nutritional decline is likely marginal at best, as the very high cooking temperatures associated with kibble production do not come into play and any loss can be easily compensated for with the addition of an appropriate vitamin/ mineral package. Additionally, some ingredients enjoy greater bioavailability when cooked, a feature missing from raw foods.

These baked diets, in my opinion, are the future of pet food; at least the near future. I anticipate they will grow significantly in popularity over the next few years. So what does one of these diets look like? Deboned chicken (breast, whole thighs), peas, pinto beans, fava beans, vegetable oil, pumpkin, apple pomace, chicken liver, chicken fat . . . (author's note: These ingredients are followed by the vitamin/mineral supplement package that I will not burden you with here. Also included is a comprehensive family of beneficial bacteria cultures such as dried lactobacillus casei fermentation product, which will improve digestion, help synthesize vitamins, and support your pet's overall health.)

The fresh chicken provided here, along with the legumes, will deliver sufficient proteins and other nutrients for your pet. While the chicken will be reduced somewhat through the cooking process, so will all of the other fresh ingredients which, being more water rich than the chicken, will ensure that quality chicken is the main ingredient going into your pet. The pumpkin, a member of the squash family, is a nutrient-rich vegetable and a great source of fiber. Apple pomace is what's left over after most of the juice has been pressed out and offers the same health benefits as eating an apple. Unlike even the best of kibble with a moisture content of about 10 percent or less, the moisture in the diet presented above comes in at 55 percent, making this baked diet much closer to a natural, healthier meal complete with added safety features compliments of the cooking process, safety features that are not characteristic of raw diets. This meal also qualifies as being low glycemic.

The ingredient list here has been created to establish a good nutritional meal for Spot. It has not been dressed up with a collection of nutritionally questionable ingredients designed to impress the paropet. Simply defrost and serve to provide your pet with a tasty, nutritious meal.

DEHYDRATED FOODS

There are some additional options for feeding your pet that fall between raw food and kibble diets. Let's look at a dehydrated dog food ingredient list: cooked free range meat (author's note: available in free-range buffalo, beef, chicken, or wild-caught salmon), naked oats, wheat germ, eggs, liver, carrots, grapefruit, winter squash, broccoli, cranberries, limes, papaya, apple, parsley, garlic, goat milk yogurt, flaxseed, cider vinegar, egg shell, olive oil. A statement on a package reads: All fruits and vegetables used in all our diets are raw and edible table-grade quality.

Dehydrated pet foods, such as grain-free kibble diets, gained in popularity in response to the objections to raw diets. You can, however, find dehydrated raw, grain-free diets in the marketplace; this product, with oats and cooked meat, isn't one of them. As with frozen diets, antioxidant preservatives such as mixed tocopherols aren't used because the dehydration is itself the preserving method. Like some of the other diets we've examined, some of these ingredients are probably included to impress paropets and may have reduced bioavailability in their raw state.

The meat is described as *cooked* on the ingredient list, meaning that it is included in the menu in an already cooked form, and so it will likely retain its position at the top of the ingredient list during the dehydration process. This will result in a good-quality meat source being the top item going into the ingredients and into your dog. Further, the manufacturer's website advises the meats they use are locally obtained as either fresh or flash frozen. It's also nice to see free-range meat sources being used, as the meat may be leaner and hopefully possess fewer chemical contaminants than might be found in meat from typical sources.

While they do use some grain products in the form of oats and wheat germ, both are superior to cheap protein fillers: in any event, this diet cannot be described as grain rich when compared with many foods. If you were stuck on a desert island, this would be an excellent diet to keep your dog—and you—going until rescuers showed up with a supply of steaks and beer.

FREEZE-DRIED FOODS

A small market niche is freeze-dried pet food products. Like dehydrated foods and grain-free kibble, freeze-dried products were developed to provide a user-friendly alternative to the inconvenience of raw diets. As ingredient lists for these diets mirror those found in the frozen and dehydrated foods presented above, we'll skip the redundancy of discussing that which we've already covered. Many of the freeze-dried foods available are raw diets and must be handled as though you were handling fresh, raw meat. If you're using any raw food, including freeze-dried, wash your hands thoroughly after contact, clean the pet's dish after each use, discard uneaten food after thirty minutes . . . and keep your small children at a distance.

The issue with selecting a healthy diet for your cat or dog is one of basic common sense. If you commence with an idea of how you would like to feed your cat or dog, then you'll hopefully be less confused by the mishmash of information that comes your way. Don't arbitrarily believe anything promoted in print or electronic advertising media. For example, I've never seen a pet food advertised on television or in print that I would feed to my dog. I often tell customers that if a company can afford great advertisements, they may not be able to afford to put good ingredients in the foods they manufacture. Thought for the day: Between the expense of national advertising campaigns and the demands of shareholders, will there be sufficient profit remaining to feed a healthy meal to your pet?

So, common sense dictates that, when shopping for a quality pet diet, you should ignore all media pitches and be skeptical of biased product information found on manufacturer's self-promoting websites. (That suggestion might also apply when shopping for your own food.) Instead, talk to the staff in pet food stores. You might get better information from smaller independent stores than from the box stores or corporate chains with their high staff turnover. Staying with a smaller store also allows staff to know and understand your pet's nutritional needs. (As a small-store owner, I confess to being prejudiced.) A word of caution: some stores, if they have a house brand, will automatically direct you toward these products. House brands in pet food stores, like house brands in supermarkets, drug stores, hardware stores, and others, are usually the most profitable products in the store. However, being a house brand should not be viewed as an automatic disqualifier. Some house brands may provide a good-quality diet; others not. Examine its merits as you would any other food. If the house brand provides both affordability and quality, buy it!

You will also find valuable information about pet foods on the Internet . . . along with a great deal of misguided views, biased opinions, and purely erroneous material: cruise the information highway with care. This point made itself obvious to us a while back. We were frustrated with a former employee who believed nearly everything she read on the Internet; if it was online, it was gospel, regardless of how suspect the information proved to be. She began passing her erroneous findings along to customers, causing confusion and poor decisions being made for their pets. This was unacceptable for us; that's why she's now a "former" employee.

That's well and good. Now that you've received input from various sources, start reading labels. Start with the ingredients label and study it carefully. Have pen and paper handy for any notes you care to take. Ask questions of the staff regarding ingredients you're unsure of. If answers aren't handy or seem suspicious, check it out on the Internet (carefully) when you get home. If you spot ingredients listed in the following section, a mental warning flag should pop up.

INGREDIENT NO-NO'S

I have given you some insight into many of the ingredients I don't like to find in a pet food. It's important to keep them in mind when reviewing any ingredient list. However, my "don't like" list includes several other undesirable ingredients; in my opinion, none of these ingredients should be approved by AAFCO for use in pet foods, but they are. The following is a brief review of those already identified, along with some others not previously mentioned.

- Unspecified (mystery) ingredients such as poultry fat, animal fat, meat meal, meat and bone meal, blood meal, poultry meal, and fish meal. If you don't know what you're buying, why buy it?
- Poor-quality meat sources, such as chicken by-products, chicken by-product meal, lamb by-products, and poultry by-product meal, and the worst of the lot, meat and bone meal. All of these may contain 4D animal sources along with other animal parts your pet doesn't need to ingest.
- Any and all food dyes. Our pets don't care about the pretty colors and don't need them. The colors are there to impress you.
- Chemical additives such as propyl gallate, glyceryl monostearate, and propylene glycol. As well as their being used in foods, beware of the latter's frequent inclusion in popular mass-market

soft, moist dog and cat treats. Hopefully, you won't find the latter, propylene glycol, in cat food products, as it has been banned for use due to feline health issues. It is time to ban its use in dog foods and treats.

- Flavor enhancers designed to mask a recipe of poor- and low-quality ingredients: digest, animal digest, all sugar sources, excessive salt (sodium chloride). Also fats such as tallow and lard—included to improve palatability—provide little nutritional value.
- Chemical preservatives such as ethoxyquin, BHA, and BHT. They are good for preserving the fats in foods but bad for preserving our pet's health. They are associated with cancers and other health issues. While often no longer listed in the ingredients, the danger is that they may be used by rendering operations supplying cheap fats and meat by-products to pet food manufacturers.
- Too much grain and too many grain sources, particularly the high-glycemic grains such as wheat, corn, and rice; cheap protein fillers such as corn gluten meal; soybean ingredients of any description; poor-quality grain sources such as brewer's rice; assorted mill runs such as soybean mill run. Some of these items are little more than floor sweepings and belong in the local landfill rather than in our pets.
- Grain fraction combinations such as corn and corn gluten meal, or rice, brewer's rice, and rice flour. The purpose here is to cut costs, deceive consumers, and nutritionally cheat our pets.
- Whey. A milk by-product; whey is a good protein source but very high in lactose. As most cats and dogs are lactose intolerant, whey can create allergies and cause vomiting and diarrhea.
- Generic terms such as *flavorings*. What are they? Forget generic! Please, tell us what you're using . . . unless you're not proud of it.
- Plasma (blood) protein. Blood is incorporated into the food as a protein source, and possibly as a flavor enhancer.
- Truly questionable ingredients such as cellulose, rice hulls, and peanut hulls. Here's Wikipedia's explanation of rice hulls: "Rice hulls are the outermost covering of the rice and come as organic rice hulls and natural rice hulls. Rice hulls are an inexpensive by-product of human food processing, serving as a source of fiber that is considered a filler ingredient in cheap pet foods."

Most cellulose used in pet foods is powdered, dry wood and provides absolutely no benefit to a cat, dog, or person that I'm aware of. It is often included in pet weight-loss diets because of its indigestibility. Why such items are allowed to be used in the manufacturing of pet foods is beyond my understanding.

As most, if not all, of these undesirable foodstuffs and chemicals are approved for inclusion in our pet foods by AAFCO, you begin to understand why I cannot respect the association's involvement in determining what is acceptable for our pets to eat. For my dog Taffy, their standards are simply insufficient. I'm concerned that foodstuffs that have been approved for livestock such as cattle, hogs, and horses are then also somehow considered acceptable for carnivores such as our cats and dogs. They don't seem to understand that my dog is not a goat or your cat a cow. Where our pets are concerned, they need to raise the bar.

The bottom line is this: as you cannot rely on organizations like AAFCO to have your pet's best interests at heart, the responsibility for providing them with a healthy diet rests directly on your shoulders. Fortunately for Spot and Whiskers, there are many quality diets from which to select that avoid the inclusion of undesirable ingredients. That being said, we all must recognize that, in spite of our best efforts to become informed consumers, there is a measure of trust on our part that the manufacturers are providing what they claim. I suspect our trust is often abused, in part because AAFCO's guidelines and policies allow the industry great leeway to do as they please.

CHAPTER 3

How to Read a Pet Food Package

The average dog is a nicer person than the average person.

—Andrew A. Rooney

Now that you've mastered the ingredient list, there is additional information on a pet food package or label that is important to understand. Knowing what this information is, and how to read and understand it, is an important step toward becoming an informed pet food shopper. Trust me on this.

Let's begin with some supergood holistic advice for you . . . read what comes next. After reading this premium information, you'll be ultrainformed where pet foods are concerned. (There's a purpose in my use of misapplied superlatives here.) What's in a word? Often, not much! Let's look at some adjectives such as *super*, *ultra*, *holistic*, and *premium*, all of which I've abused at the beginning of this paragraph. Manufacturers often use these and other exaggerating descriptors to describe their pet foods. Let's think about this for a moment. Do you prefer to feed Whiskers a dish of cat food, or a dish of *premium* cat food? As Whiskers can't read (my assumption) and isn't likely making the purchase decision anyway (another assumption), and as you love your cat, you'd probably opt for the *premium* cat food. *Premium* means it has to be a better-quality diet, right? Well then, why not move up the food chain another step and buy a bag of *super premium* cat food? You can't go wrong with that, can you? Clearly, *super premium* is superior to staid old *premium*. Or, even better, step up again and buy Whiskers a bag of *ultra premium* cat food. You can't top *ultra*! These are my exaggerations here, but, following that line of thought, a bag of *ultra super premium* cat food has to be as good as it gets, right?

Wrong! Commencing a couple of decades ago, we humans became increasingly interested in improving our diets. Food marketers quickly discovered the magic associated with the word *holistic*, which soon began appearing everywhere, including on packages of our pet diets. So now, nothing can improve on a bag of *ultra super premium holistic* cat food (sarcastically exaggerated to make a point). Recall, please, my earlier assumption that your cat can't read; those descriptors are prominently displayed on the package to impress you. Your dog or cat doesn't care. While the marketing managers who create the packaging love such inviting, seductive adjectives, they are as empty of meaning as Wall Street is of ethics.

To date, for pet foods, I believe *holistic* remains the king of quality-exaggerating adjectives, a wonderful word that too often fails to deliver on its enticing promise. If *holistic* is under threat at all, it's from *organic*; *organic* is making slow progress in penetrating the pet food world, possibly due to the fact that marketing managers are handicapped by legal definitions tied to the word. Another favorite is "natural." "Natural" is so desirable it's even incorporated into some brand names. Natural suggests all the wholesome goodness Mother Nature provides. Don't be deceived; cancer and E. coli are also natural.

In the first paragraph at the beginning of this chapter I suggested you trust me. Here's my point. When reading information on pet food packaging, place your trust in a safe location and drag out your skepticism; skepticism will better serve you here than will trust. Words such as *premium*, *ultra*, and *holistic* are powerful lures, promises of a quality level too often undelivered in terms of your pet's nutrition. Don't be fooled by their use on a package of pet (or human) food. There are no protective laws governing the use of such adjectives by food manufacturers for describing the diets they want you to buy. Bluntly stated, a pet food manufacturer can package the absolute lowest quality pet food ever produced and legally label it as *ultra* or *super* or *premium* or *holistic* pet food, or use any of the descriptors in whatever combination they prefer; for example, Uncle Dave's Super Ultra Holistic Premium Dog Food.

Remember, if you're not an informed consumer you could be an uninformed dupe. Don't be seduced by inane superlatives.

ALL LIFE STAGES

There is no psychiatrist in the world like a puppy licking your face.

—Ben Williams

Packages of pet food can display other interesting tidbits of information. One term appearing today with increasing frequency, but usually only on better-quality diets, is *All Life Stages Diet* (or similar wording). To properly explain this, we need to briefly revisit the history of pet foods.

Recall that, for much of the pet food industry's life, products were primarily built from the waste generated by the production of human foods. The wastes (or more nicely phrased when used in pet foods, by-products) are nutritionally inferior ingredients because many of their nutrients are stripped from them during the process that creates them. For adult dogs and cats, nutritional demands are usually less than that of growing kittens and puppies or pregnant/nursing mothers. In order to ensure that the young animals received adequate nutrition, the manufacturers were obligated to develop kitten and puppy formulas, formulas that usually contained an increase in the meat content along with a boost in the vitamin/mineral supplement package added to the food. For that, they often charged you more. Once the animal became a young adult, it could be weaned off the meatier, expensive diet and put on the less expensive adult formula.

With the introduction of superior quality diets, the need for kitten and puppy formulas—if eating these improved diets—pretty much vanished. Both the younger pet and the adult were now receiving the healthy nutrition they required from the same diet. On these new diets, rather than creating puppy/kitten formulas, it really boils down to how much food is required for a meal. A growing kitten or puppy, energetic and constantly active, simply needs more food when the quality of the food is adequate in the first place (versus providing a better food if the quality is inadequate). In this case it's the quality of the food that dictates the quantity of food required for adequate nutrition. A mature, more sedate pet will survive nicely with less food.

The problem the producers of better-quality diets ran into, however, was one of consumer expectations. For decades we had become ac-customed to the fact that we required puppy food for puppies, kitten food for kittens, and other formulas for adults and seniors. A food that covered adult, juvenile, and senior was met with skepticism by many customers, and still is today. It's slowly changing, as more customers understand the benefits associated with superior diets. Natura Pet, for example, went for years without providing a puppy formula in their Innova line. They finally introduced a puppy line for no other reason, I suspect, than the need to conform to customer expectations. The puppies didn't really need it as Natura's adult formula sufficed for both juvenile and adult life stages.

Today you will still find kitten and puppy formulas in those foods of questionable quality. For those diets, it remains a necessity to ensure your four-footed youngsters get off to a good start in life. You will discover that producers of high-quality diets have taken one of two options. They will either produce kitten/puppy diets separate from their adult formulas, or more sensibly from my point of view, market their products as All Life Stages.

CALORIE CONTENT

> No heaven will not ever Heaven be; unless my cats are there to welcome me.
>
> —Anonymous

This information has started appearing on pet food packages in recent years. It's a handy piece of information to know, particularly if your pet is overweight and you have to control the amount of calories your pet is receiving. The amount of calories/cup in most pet foods will typically range from a low of around three hundred for a diet food to an upper range of five hundred and up for a performance food. The two examples provided below are from a dog and cat food, both grain free and from the same manufacturer:

Dog: 3,719 kcals/kg (370 kcals/cup) calculated metabolized energy

Cat: 3,745 kcals/kg (390 kcals/cup) calculated metabolized energy

What is metabolized energy (ME)? Basically, metabolized energy is the kcal energy as shown on the package. It represents the amount of energy provided to your pet by the food during the digestion process. Food material not metabolized ends up mostly as digestive gases, feces, and urine, and it is passed from the body. The calculated amount of energy going into the pet, less the material not metabolized, becomes the formula for determining the ME.

Breed, age, sex, lifestyle, health, and other factors all are requirements in determining the amount of calories each pet requires on a daily basis. As every pet is different, and as the package information is a calculation, the package information should be considered as a guide, not a hard number.

The ME information on the package can also be an indicator of the quality of the food. The higher the ME value, the greater the caloric density of the food in the same way that a piece of an energy bar the size of a soda cracker will pack in more caloric energy than a soda cracker. The benefit of a denser food to you, the consumer, is that you should require less food on a daily basis to feed Spot or Whiskers than if using a food with a lower ME value. A side benefit here is that you should have less waste being generated in the form of urine and feces. When cleaning up the litter box or backyard, stools should be firmer and smaller.

The calorie content is at best a generalized guide. The caloric information provided is the result of a mathematical calculation, the accuracy of which leaves something to be desired. Just to confuse matters even more, it should be noted that the ME in denser foods may be understated, while those in less-dense foods will be overstated with the math formula used. This can lead to confusion as a less-dense, grain-rich diet might in some cases provide an ME similar to that of a better-quality diet; in short, information that is mathematically calculated from arbitrarily estimated or assigned values can possibly be massaged to provide a desired result. They wouldn't do that . . . would they? If suspicious, return to the ingredient list for insight.

Use this calorie content information as a guide, but don't make a buying decision based solely on it.

AAFCO STATEMENT

I wonder if other dogs think poodles are members of a weird religious cult.

—Rita Rudner

Your packaging will contain an AAFCO statement. The statement identifies how the nutritional adequacy was determined and for which life stage or lifestyle the product was approved. AAFCO regulations require that the manufacturer be able to substantiate the statement, and it provides three methods for compliance (www.petfood.aafco.org/caloriecontent.aspx).

1. Laboratory analysis: The finished product is compared to minimum nutritional values established by the AAFCO Nutrient Profiles for dogs or cats. The label on the package will state: "XYZ Dog/Cat Food is formulated to meet the nutritional levels established by the AAFCO Dog/Cat Food Nutrient Profiles for (appropriate life stage)." This means that a nutrition profile for felines and canines has been determined by one or more dog/cat nutrition experts, and the food is fine for our pets as long as it meets the established requirements.

2. Feeding trials: The finished product that has been laboratory tested is fed to dogs or cats according to established AAFCO protocols. The label on the package states: "Animal feeding tests using AAFCO procedures substantiate that XYZ Dog/Cat Food provides complete and balanced nutrition for (appropriate life stage)."

What's a feeding trial? AAFCO feeding trial standards for pet food manufacturers requires that six out of eight animals complete a twenty-six-week feeding trial without showing clinical or pathological signs of nutritional deficiency or excess. The overall health of the cats and dogs involved in the trial is evaluated by a veterinarian before and after the test (and probably during). Four blood values measured after the trial and the average values of the test subjects must meet minimum levels. Participating animals are not allowed to lose more than 15 percent of their starting weight.

That's it in a nutshell. These feeding trials have long been a source of contention for paropets. I assume the feeding supervisors only select very robust animals for these trials; I certainly would if I was in their shoes. There's an additional concern regarding impartiality. These trials are usually conducted by in-house researchers or consulting veterinarians/nutritionists. Good results allow staff to retain their jobs and consultants to enjoy future contracts. And the trial is only for six months. If two animals (25 percent) in the trial actually die or do poorly on the food, the product is still considered safe for our pets as long as the remaining animals make it to the end and pass the evaluations. Sadly, there's no way of determining the product's shortcomings if fed on a longer-term basis. After the six-month period has been completed, it's our pets that become their guinea pigs. If they were testing foods to be fed to their own children rather than our pets, one wonders if the trial process might be longer and more thorough.

3. Analysis comparable in nutritional adequacy: Laboratory analysis of the finished product is compared with nutritional values from a similar product fed to dogs and cats according to AAFCO protocols. The label on the package states: "XYZ Dog/Cat Food provides complete and balanced nutrition for (appropriate life stage) and is comparable in nutritional adequacy to a product which has been substantiated using AAFCO feeding tests." This relates to items #1 and #2 above. It means that if I'm making a new product, Food B, and it's very similar to an existing product, Food A, which has already been approved under either of the above protocols, then it's safe to assume that Food B is suitable for pets to eat.

The manufacturer is required to include the AAFCO statement on the package. In my opinion the statement's real purpose is to present you, the consumer, with a feeling of comfort and the impression of creditability. I don't believe AAFCO provides much in the way of a benefit to our cats and dogs, as noted elsewhere, and I don't see this statement as having much relevance for you or your pets.

BEST BEFORE DATE

> You can say any foolish thing to a dog, and the dog will give you a look that says, "My God, you're right! I never would've thought of that!"
>
> —Dave Barry

Along with the ingredient list, the best before date is an important piece of information. I consider it to be a customer MUST READ. It must be displayed on every package of kibble or can of food. On cans, you'll usually find it stamped on the top lid or bottom of the can. On bags, the date can be difficult to locate, as there is often no in-your-face location that's readily available. It's up to the whim of each manufacturer. Some make it easy; others make it a challenge. In fact, a manufacturer might well have it in a different location every time they run a batch of food. Even I have been forced to spend a couple of minutes scanning a bag to locate the date to satisfy a customer's query. I've also performed this frustrating search when buying perishable packaged food for my own table. Why do some of these food producers make it a challenge to find such a valuable piece of information?

Food retailers should be rotating their inventory with every incoming shipment to ensure their customers are receiving the freshest product available. Don't count on this happening. Some retailers or their staff might be sloppy, indifferent, or just plain lazy.

Sometimes it can be difficult for the retailer to catch errors made by others. Manufacturers and wholesalers, like retailers, should be rotating the inventory in their warehouses. While it doesn't happen often, we have received foods from time to time that have almost no shelf life left on the package, and a few times where the food has actually expired. In other cases, food being received into inventory is older than the food we already have on our shelves. It happens! I'm certain most retailers and wholesalers conscientiously make an effort to keep their supplies fresh. You, the consumer, also need to be alert by checking every can or bag before you part with your money.

Canned diets, because they're normally cooked in a sealed can, like canned salmon at your supermarket, have a much longer shelf life than do dry foods. Most canned products will show upward of three years of shelf life. For dry foods, expect to see a shelf life from six to fifteen months. For frozen diets, it's very important to check the best before date on the package, as the shelf life is often dictated by the quality of the packaging and the efficiency of the freezers it has been stored in prior to your purchase.

How old is too old? I'm comfortable with using canned foods right up to the expiry date on the lid. Even up to two or three months beyond the expiry date wouldn't bother me. Mind you, I'm talking about what I would use, not what I would sell. I wouldn't sell any canned food with less than three month's expiry remaining, and prior to that, I would probably put anything on sale to clear out my aging inventory.

Dry food is a different conversation. We pull anything from our shelves that has only two months of shelf life remaining before reaching its expiry date. I would suggest that, as a concerned consumer, you not purchase any dry food that has less than two months of shelf life remaining. If I was intent on buying it anyway, I'd push the retailer for a discount. If you can't use the bag of food up within four or five weeks I recommend not buying it. Dig out a fresh bag, if available. Some manufacturers include the date the food was produced on the package. They all should do that: whenever possible, purchase food that's no more than six months old for maximum nutritional benefits. The older a food becomes, the less nutritionally beneficial it will be for Whiskers or Spot. While it's beneficial for manufacturers and distributors to have expiry dates of a year or more following production, I suspect the food is only at its best for about six months.

If you're tempted to purchase pet food from nontraditional sources, such as clearance stores, bulk stores, online stores, discount stores, dollar stores, and flea markets, I suggest you carefully look at the best before date on the package. Otherwise, you and your pet may be in for an unpleasant surprise. I'd also recommend you check the bag for puncture damage prior to making the purchase. If punctured, the best before date becomes meaningless. Sometimes, a good deal is a bad deal.

All it takes is a couple of seconds to check the best before date. It's time well spent.

FEEDING GUIDE

> The greatness of a nation and its moral progress can be judged by the way its animals are treated.
>
> —Mahatma Gandhi

Along with the ingredient list, the feeding guide represents some of the more useful information found on the package. The key word to remember here is *guide*. The manufacturer knows nothing about your pet's physical condition, age, or lifestyle (such as whether it receives one walk a day or one a week, or if the walk lasts for fifteen minutes or an hour). They know nothing regarding the state of your pet's health, or if it's a fussy eater or a glutton, or if you supplement its diet with other foods. That's why it's called a feeding guide, not a feeding regulation or feeding rule. You're the one who knows all of those things about your cat or dog. You're the one responsible for feeding your pet appropriately.

The best feeding guides will commence with the pet's weight in pounds and/or kilograms and then chart out a series of age stages from weeks or months to adult. Some will also include additional feeding information based on specific conditions; such as active or inactive, pregnant or lactating. Read it all, keeping in mind it is but a guide.

As an example, a fifty-pound, eight-month-old dog might require three cups of food a day. An adult fifty-pound dog on the same food might only require two cups a day. Taffy, as a thirty-pound senior, receives approximately two-thirds of a cup of food twice daily (plus everything she can mooch in between). If her weight increases a bit, the food decreases. If she gets a bit thin, the food increases. In spite of her gluttonous tendency, her weight variation at her annual checkups has usually remained within a pound or two.

Like the calorie content information, the feeding guide can also be used as a measure of the quality of the food. There are grain-rich diets that require four or more cups of food to be fed daily to a fifty-pound dog, rather than the approximate two cups for denser foods. If that is what you're feeding, I can only hope you purchase your poop bags in bulk.

Tip: Like the calorie content information, the feeding guide can be important in determining value for you. If you have two foods, each in five-pound bags, and both with similar price tags, the denser formula, requiring less food per serving, will provide better value for you as long as the quality of ingredients are equal.

Finally, it should come as no surprise to learn that, generally speaking, the recommendations on most package feeding guides are on the "generous side." Gosh, what a shocker!

GUARANTEED ANALYSIS

I've met many thinkers and many cats, but the wisdom of cats is infinitely superior.

—Hippolyte Taine

Where package information is concerned, we've arrived at the final step toward you becoming an informed consumer capable of defending yourself against both marketing sharks and inadequate government regulations. The last label you need to look at on your pet's food is the guaranteed analysis (GA), found on packages of frozen, dry, or canned pet products. Look at it . . . but don't spend a lot of time studying it.

It's always been interesting to me that people who see themselves as being well-informed on pet food matters, such as breeders, trainers, and serious pet people, go straight to the GA information on the package, sometimes to the exclusion of all other information. They study the GA carefully, and make buying decisions based on it. I don't understand that level of interest in the GA because, from my point of view, it represents some of the most useless information on the package. Here's why. The guaranteed analysis provides the appearance of giving you valuable information while at the same time providing you with very little in the way of useable facts. What a clever (and legal) deception! The GA provides facts without substance, or may I say facts without factuality. Let's analyze a typical GA to see what I'm talking about.

Guaranteed Analysis
Crude Protein, Not less than (or minimum) 22.0%
Crude Fat, Not less than (or minimum) 12.0%
Crude Fiber, Not more than (or maximum) 4.0%
Moisture, Not more than (or maximum) 11.0%

I've arbitrarily drawn a line under the *moisture* information, as everything above the line is, for the most part, standard on all packages. Most GA charts will contain additional information of little real relevance to you, the reader, or, to put it another way, the information below the line will be as irrelevant as the information above the line. But hey . . . it all looks good! For example, of the two bags of dog food I have in the house, one lists additional values (below my arbitrary line), for zinc, selenium, vitamin E, and omega-6 and 3 fatty acids, in that order. The other bag lists, in order, copper, manganese, zinc, vitamins A and E, taurine, and omega-3 and 6 fatty acids. Other products will provide similar information. The omegas and taurine are asterisked, with the addition of this proviso: *Not recognized as an essential nutrient by the AAFCO dog food nutrient profile.* All of these additional items are provided with minimum or maximum values.

My objection, as noted above, is that there's no hard information to be found here. Take the first item as an example, crude protein, minimum 22 percent. What the heck does *minimum* mean? I'm exaggerating here by asking: is the protein content 22 percent, or maybe 32 percent? Who knows? Maybe a lab rat somewhere is in the know, but the rest of us remain in the dark! We're parked in an information void when it comes to knowing the actual protein content of this food. In fairness, the regulatory authorities require the manufacturers to ensure that their product is "close" to the values they provide in the GA. As consumers, we're left wondering, how close is close?

The same lack of information is relative to all of the other values, regardless of whether they're listed as *minimum/maximum* or *not more/ less than*. For consumers, there is little value to be found in these values. They're included on the package information because, by AAFCO regulation, their inclusion is a requirement. Perhaps it's time for AAFCO and the pet food industry to revisit the guaranteed analysis with the intention of tightening up the information provided. Pet parents everywhere would appreciate it. You don't normally see these vague values on packages of human foods, so obviously it's doable.

Looking again at the crude protein, the real issue isn't the percentage of protein; it's the quality of the protein sources that is important. The GA tells us nothing regarding the quality. You can generate a suitable protein reading for the GA by using ground-up leather from old shoes and chopped-up hair from the nearest barbershop (hair is primarily protein). Have a laboratory analyze the leather/hair mixture for protein and you'll be rewarded with an acceptable crude protein value. That's all it takes! As you might imagine, while providing a suitable protein rating, hair and shoe leather are pretty much indigestible, even in an acidic environment such as your pet's gut, thus making those ingredients nutritionally valueless. If you doubt hair's digestibility, ask a cat parent about hairballs. Feathers are also indigestible . . . and dangerous. A breeder once came into my store looking for a better food. Her interest was the result of a nasty stab wound on her hand, received when she reached into a bag of food and ended up with a piece of sharp quill imbedded in her palm. When she complained to the company, they sent her some coupons for more of their cheap food. Rather than coupons, they should include a supply of bandages in every bag.

This goes to the issue of protein fillers in pet foods, such as corn gluten meal. The protein in corn gluten meal, while more digestible than shoe leather and hair, isn't well digested by cats or dogs. It does look like food on the ingredient list to those who don't understand what they're looking at, if they even bother reading the IL, but it isn't a good source of nutrition for your pet. That's why we refer to it as a "protein filler" or just "filler," as it supports a suitable protein rating for the GA while contributing little to your pet's nutritional welfare.

Don't spend too much time studying the GA.

In summary, I maintain the most valuable information available to the consumer on a package of pet food is that provided by the ingredient list (IL). While the IL doesn't tell you everything you need to know, at the very least it tells you what's in the package, and if you understand what you're reading, it also provides a reasonable guide as to the quantity and quality of the ingredients. As mentioned previously, the ingredient list is the first information on the package that I study when determining if the product is suitable for use with my dog and for the loved pets of my customers.

WHAT'S MISSING FROM THE GA?

It's fine that the GA provides us with information (in a lame manner) regarding protein, fat, and more, but we're never provided even a clue as to the carbohydrate content of the diet. Why not? Your guess is as good as mine. I suspect it has to do with the fact that, when the rules were being made, it didn't serve the interests of those companies providing grain-rich diets to have you thinking about how many carbohydrates were actually being fed to Whiskers and Spot; having to list the ingredients was probably all the trauma they could cope with. Carbohydrate values are an important piece of information. In food terms, carbohydrates usually refer to complex carbohydrates (starch) and simple carbohydrates (sugar).

Fortunately, there's a simple calculation you can use to determine the carbohydrate content of the food you are feeding to your pet. You would be wise to do the calculation, as the result may surprise you. The complete contents of any pet food must total 100 percent, so 100 percent is your starting point. From that, subtract the percentages shown for each ingredient on the GA (except the fiber, as fiber is already considered a carbohydrate). Also, if the ash (mineral) content is not listed, you will have to allow from 5 percent to 8 percent for it in your calculations (I'm using 8 percent here). So, using the GA example in the section above, plus an allowance for ash, you would calculate the carbohydrate content as: Out of 100 percent, 22 percent is protein, 12 percent is fat, 11 percent is moisture, and 8 percent is ash, which means 47 percent of the food consists of carbohydrates.

Where protein content is high, carbohydrate content will be low. Why is this important? Remember, your cats and dogs, being carnivores, will be healthier with protein than with carbs, as carbs are more likely to influence issues such as excess weight and diabetes.

FOOD SUPPLIERS

Now that you know what to look for in pet food ingredients and understand the information provided on the packaging, some consideration should be given regarding where you shop. It shouldn't be a casual decision. You can find pet foods for sale everywhere from the convenience store on a nearby corner to the pet supply box store across town. Where you shop is important both for your pocketbook and for Spot's and Whiskers's nutritional needs, and it depends a great deal on what you expect from your supplier.

Initially, most pet foods were primarily sold through grocery store channels, which is understandable in that almost all pet food products were produced by manufacturers of human foods or companies associated with them, and who, through their various arrangements, were well connected with the established grocery supply chain. Feed supply stores were (and still are) also used as pet food outlets. Eventually, small, independent pet supply stores began appearing, specializing in products for pets only, such as food, accessories, bedding, and pet shampoos. Some also sold a variety of live pets, providing everything from puppies to piranhas.

Some independent stores eventually morphed into chains of small stores: chains enjoy greater buying and marketing power. Some chains are corporately owned while others are franchise operations. Eventually, large box stores appeared on the scene. Most box store operations are corporate chains. Most recently, online stores have sprung up, taking advantage of the growing popularity of Internet shopping.

As the owner of a small, franchised pet supply store, I confess to a healthy bias favoring my style of business. However, even I am forced to admit there's a long list of both pros and cons for each player in the game. When seeking the ideal pet food supplier to service your needs, there are four main points to consider: product selection, product knowledge, pet knowledge, and service. Each of them is important, and each of them can influence the nutritional health of Whiskers and Spot. Here's an example of bad service I experienced in a local competitor's store.

A few years back I visited a nearby competitor to indulge in a bit of snooping: it's a corporate chain store. It was early evening, and the store was quiet, just me and one employee. The employee was in his late teens, and when I entered the store he was standing by the cash counter busily bouncing a hard rubber ball on the floor, probably a dog toy from off their shelf. Thump, thump, thump! He was too busy with the ball to even make eye contact with me as I entered the store.

I wandered up and down the aisles, often out of his sight for several minutes. He had no idea what I was doing, but I knew where he was and what he was doing. Thump, thump, thump! He was so dedicated to that ball game you would think he was going after a Guinness record. Snooping mission completed, and as I had my hand on the door to leave, he stopped bouncing the ball long enough to ask if I required any assistance. I shook my head no and continued out the door. I could hear the thump, thump, thump resume as the door slowly closed behind me. That young man was no asset to his employer, but, with such poor service, I considered him to be a wonderful asset for my store, located only a few blocks distant. As I drove away, I was wishing they would promote him to manager and put him on duty sixty hours a week. Thump, thump, thump! Why would any consumer give their business to a merchant providing such poor service?

So, yes, while service is important, there are also other options for you to consider. It would be a mistake to assume all pet food suppliers are equal. Where you shop depends on the quality of products you want and the level of service you desire. If you wish for a more personalized relationship providing support and advice regarding Whiskers or Spot, shop around until you find the business capable of providing it. It may prove to be one of the most beneficial relationships you and your cat or dog ever develop. Here are your options:

Supermarkets/Grocery: Due to convenience, these outlets sell large volumes of pet food, both dry and canned, and some related supplies such as litter. Many have devoted a great deal of shelf space to what, for them, is a profitable item, often more profitable than many of the human foods they sell. Generally, the foods available here are those that are the less expensive, grain-based diets, as these are usually the more profitable lines, lines that enjoy significant marketing support from the manufacturer, including co-op advertising ventures. Selection, even within a line, is usually limited, governed by consumer demand. Prices here are usually comparable to those found in their surrounding marketplace. Advice on your pet's nutrition is not available.

Mixed Merchandisers: These are the Walmarts, Targets, and their kin. This group is rapidly expanding their selections of pet foods and accessories, as they realize pet supplies, a category formerly all but ignored, will grow their businesses and their profits. They offer a wider selection of products than that found in supermarkets but, for the most part, they are still focused on products made popular through extensive media advertising by the manufacturer. If they have a house brand of pet food, there will be a larger selection of this line available, but the wise shopper will take pains to investigate the ingredient profile of that food. Prices can be at or below those found in the surrounding marketplace, and advertised specials are frequently used to draw you into the store. Advice on your pet's nutritional needs is not available.

Pet Supply Box Stores: This group probably has the most to lose as the mixed merchandisers continue expanding their offerings in the pet category. The major advantage provided by these box stores is selection. With their large square footage devoted solely to pets and pet supplies, it's impossible for smaller stores to compete when it comes to selection. Low prices are often provided for the first year or two of operation to drive out competition, but eventually their pricing seems to creep up to marketplace standards. Some food manufacturers represented in these stores—having learned to their chagrin that price cutting on their products is detrimental to their overall sales and reputations—have agreements in place to prevent their products from being used as loss leaders by box stores. Box-store pricing for related services such as grooming or training can be at or higher than those in the surrounding community. While their original focus was on food lines that were heavily supported by manufacturer advertising, efforts have been made in recent years to improve their selection with the addition of better-quality diets. They will have a house brand of pet food; you should investigate the ingredient profile of the diet. Advice on your pet's nutritional needs in box stores can be hit and miss as the staff turnover in these stores is often sufficiently high as to be detrimental to acquiring good product/pet knowledge.

Online Suppliers: When these businesses first began appearing, visionaries predicted brick-and-mortar stores like mine were all but doomed, fated to go the way of the dinosaurs. The seers need to revisit their tea leaves, as that hasn't happened. Due to the high costs associated with shipping large, heavy bags of pet food, and the precautions needed to ensure you don't run out of food (resulting in having a hungry cat or dog eating emergency rations for a few days), online food shopping failed to reach its potential. However, online stores are good sources for pet accessories, especially items that are unique and all but impossible for traditional stores to carry due to limited demand. Returning products can be a nuisance. If buying food here, advice on your pet's nutrition can be hit or miss, depending largely on the knowledge and experience of those running the business.

Small Stores—Corporate-Owned Chains: These chain-store operations can be large, over fifty stores, or small, with only three or four stores. The quality of knowledge and service can vary widely from one location to another as, like box stores, they often experience a high staff turnover. Product selection usually follows a cookie-cutter model, with most of their supplies sourced from a corporate-controlled distribution center. Product pricing is also centrally controlled and normally reflects average market prices, with sales events and special offers dictated by a head-office marketing department. If visiting the store for the first time, I would do a walk-through to get a feel for the type of foods they carry. Asking an employee for some advice on feeding your pet may help you in determining the service you might expect here, as well as the employee's knowledge of their own products and interest in your pet. If the chain is large enough they may have their own house brand of pet food. One of these stores was the source for the rubber ball anecdote provided earlier.

Small Stores—Franchise Chains: Similar in many regards to those discussed immediately above, these operations provide a significant difference. The franchisee is usually also the operator as well as the owner. As such, he/she will have more influence over the product selection and a vested interest in providing good service. Product knowledge and advice will likely be better than, or at least as good as, any you can find in your community. Pricing will likely be competitive with that in the surrounding community for the same products. If you become a frequent shopper, you may be able to negotiate a discount or other favors. Also, because the retailer/customer relationship has a chance to develop, they will come to know more about your pet, thus becoming better positioned to serve its health and nutrition needs.

Small Stores—Independents: These will be similar to that discussed immediately above. Pricing may or may not be as favorable as their competitors' pricing (chain discounts not available). Customer service levels should be high, along with product knowledge. Ask for some advice from an employee to determine both.

Veterinary Clinics: Veterinarians sell a great deal of pet food, enough to be taken seriously as competitors by all other pet food retailers. Fortunately for businesses such as mine, most vets haven't moved from the traditional grain-based diets popular decades ago. The pet food industry giants provide these diets to the vet community, and, as they are highly profitable for both vet and manufacturer, there's little incentive to change. While some products similar to those purchased from your vet can be found locally, often for significantly less money, other vet food offerings are specialty diets, designed to support specific health issues such as renal problems. One downside to shopping for food from your vet is similar to that with online stores . . . do not run out of food when the clinic is closed. Other than the specialty vet diets, you will probably find greater convenience and better-quality foods at lower prices almost everywhere else in your community. Surprisingly, you may also find better nutrition information elsewhere in your community, as nutrition knowledge is not a forte for most medical professionals such as doctors and veterinarians.

For Whiskers's or Spot's nutritional health, knowing where to shop may be almost as important as knowing what to shop for.

CHAPTER 4

More about Food

A dog teaches a boy fidelity, perseverance, and to turn around three
times before lying down.

—Robert Benchley

While knowing where to purchase pet food is important for the health
of both pet and pocketbook, there are additional factors regarding pet
food that are important to know. Here are a few that consistently come
up in conversations with my customers.

BIG DOG, LITTLE DOG

While this topic is about canine formulas, it is also applicable, in a
lesser degree, with feline foods. As discussed earlier, the better-quality
diets can be fed to juveniles . . . and adult or senior pets. There is no
need to separate adult diets from those of the juveniles unless the quality of the adult diet is insufficient to meet the nutritional needs of a
younger, growing animal.

In a similar vein, we have the issue of small- and large-breed dog
food formulas. Again, this appears to be more about marketing than it
does about your dog's nutrition. I believe it commenced years ago with
a company that put out a diet specific for dog groupings: herding dogs,
retrievers, terriers, and others. Their premise was that each of these
canine families had differing nutritional requirements. Yeah, sure!
While the formulas did in fact vary one from the other, only a certi-
fied optimist, upon contemplating the differences—which were minor

at best—would conclude that each diet was essential to each group of dogs. I don't know if I'm a skeptic or just sensible, but I failed to see any variations in those diets that would make any difference to a dog. While that line of foods didn't really gain any traction with consumers, I believe the concept evolved into something that has found a sizeable niche in today's market—foods for large dog breeds, small breeds, even medium and giant breeds.

Personally, I see all of these variations as being clever ploys to sell dog food, not to improve your dog's nutrition or lifestyle in any way. In retail, there's a marketing concept called *line extensions*. Line extensions are used by companies providing products to the retail industry to enhance their presence on the retailer's shelf. In dog food, for example, you start out with a chicken and rice adult formula, and another of the same formula for senior dogs. That's two products with maybe three bag sizes for each, which we'd refer to as three skus (stock keeping units, pronounced skuze). So, that's six skus. Fine so far! Next year you introduce a lamb formula, also in three bag sizes. A year later you show up at the retailer's door with fish formula, and six months later you're back knocking on the retailer's door with a small- and/or large-breed version of the original adult formula. And each of these new formulas comes in at least three package sizes. It's a similar story when you get into their canned food variations. These are all line extensions in that you start the line with one or two products, then keep adding versions of the original item. While the industry giants do this best, all pet food manufacturers are players in this game.

For a great example of line extensions, check out the soup display or cereal section the next time you visit your supermarket. Instead of one mushroom soup, there are often two or more variations of mushroom soup. Or you can find tomato soup beside low-salt tomato soup parked beside tomato and rice soup. Cheerios, which used to be a single product, now has a variety of flavors and package sizes from which to choose. Line extensions one and all! There are two goals here. One: to provide you, the consumer, with additional ways to spend your money on their products. Two: take up more space on the retailers' shelves for their products, thus making less space available for competitors' products. For pet foods, in none of these scenarios is your pet a part of the conversation; it's all about what's good for the manufacturer.

When I compare these small- and large-breed formulas with the original adult formula, I fail to see a change that will make any difference to a dog, regardless of the dog's size. Yes, in some large-breed formulas they include some glucosamine and chondroitin for joint health (as though small breeds don't get arthritis later in life), and the small-breed formulas are often produced with a smaller kibble size. Still, a Jack Russell can eat a large-breed food, and a Great Dane can chow down on a small-breed formula; both will do just fine nutritionally. It's all about marketing, not pet nutrition or health.

Kibble size? Customers have told me their small dog must have small kibble because it can't eat anything too large. Ironically, the same customer will buy a bag of treat biscuits for their pet, biscuits that are several times the size of a piece of kibble and which presumably their dog has no problem devouring. I'm forced to smile as they head for their car.

Other line extensions include specialty items such as dental and weight-control diets. We'll discuss weight management as a topic later. While weight-control diets continue to be popular (some are combined as senior/weight control), the dental diets seem not to have established a significant following among consumers . . . probably because they seem ineffective. A starch-rich diet from grains or potatoes is likely to cause oral problems regardless of how large you formulate the kibble. Having to chew on a large piece of kibble will probably achieve nothing. Are your teeth noticeably cleaner after eating a few crackers?

While the focus for much of this marketing activity involves dog foods, our cats have not escaped the marketer's attention. Feline line extensions include hairball, indoor cat, outdoor cat, senior cat, fat cat, and allergic cat formulas. Some companies have attempted to introduce formulas for Persians, Siamese, and others. I'm disappointed that cats failed to remain aloofly above this fray; I expected better of them. Often these specialty formulas come with a slightly higher price tag. Save your money!

Again, these things have almost everything to do with marketing and little to do with the health requirements of Whiskers and Spot.

STORING PET FOOD

It's a mystery to me that well-intentioned paropets concerned with the health of their four-footed family member, and who are willing to purchase an expensive quality diet for their pet, will then take that food home and thoughtlessly transfer it from the manufacturer's package into another container. I am, of course, discussing the storage of kibble here.

Over the years I have been surprised at the assortment of containers people use for storing pet food; containers such as large plastic trash bins, or various plastic, metal, and wood boxes. They'll use pretty much anything that comes to hand, which is perceived to be more convenient than the package they brought home from the store. It makes me shudder. There are two things that can go seriously wrong for your pet food in this situation.

Your first enemy is oxidation. Plain old air is the guilty party here. If you recall, the preservatives added to foods, such as mixed tocopherols, are to prevent the fats in the foods from turning rancid from oxidation. That's why the preservatives used are antioxidants. Once you open the package, the clock starts ticking, counting down to when the food will turn bad. If not used in a reasonable time (more on this shortly), the food will turn rancid, become unfit to eat, and quite possibly endanger your pet's health.

If you retain the food in its original package, you can reduce the amount of air in the bag by resealing it if it has a zipper lock, or using a clip of some type if not zip-locked. (The clips sold for sealing bags of potato chips are ideal.) Plastic containers are of particular concern to me. Where food storage is concerned, all plastic containers are not equal. I can't recall how many times my customers have been unable to tell me if the container they use for storing their pet's food is made of food-grade plastic or plastic created for another purpose. The problem is this: the fats in the food are acidic (fatty acid). All plastic is made from chemicals. The chemicals used in nonfood grade containers can be toxic. Some fatty acids can react to the toxic chemicals and slowly leach chemicals from the plastic directly into the food. Now your cat or dog is eating—every day—a meal laced with toxic, and probably carcinogenic, chemicals. Not good!

My advice is this: rather than decanting the food into a storage container, put the whole package into the container (after first wiping it down with a disinfectant to eliminate any dirt or contaminants that may be on the package's exterior). The packaging will protect the food from contact with the plastic and help reduce the amount of air coming into contact with the food. Still, this option is not ideal, as some plastics emit toxic gases. Ensure that the container is made of food-grade plastic; if not, don't use it. Or forget the container and leave the food in its original packaging. I'm also uncomfortable with containers made of metal or other materials. At the very least, I recommend leaving the food in its package and placing it all in the container.

Regardless of what container is used, food should not be stored in a location that is too warm or humid, as heat and moisture will hasten the deterioration of your pet's meals. Store the food in a location that's reasonably cool (room temperature in an air-conditioned home). Uncovered and unsealed concrete basement floors are less than ideal, as they often allow ground moisture to work its way to the concrete's surface. I had a customer tell me he'd purchased several bags of wild bird feed on sale and stored them on the floor of his garage. Within a few weeks the birds rejected the food, as it had turned moldy from moisture. Formerly, he only purchased one bag at a time, using it up before moisture could cause a problem. He was forced to throw out over half of his bargain bird feed, which, because of poor storage, proved to be no bargain at all.

At the end of the day remember you are storing food. Treat your pet's food as you would your own.

PET SIZE, BAG SIZE

Another way in which some customers amaze me relates to decisions regarding the size of the bag of pet food they intend to purchase. Customers will carefully evaluate the various diets in the store and ultimately select one that fits their pocketbook and quality concerns. Then, in order to get the best bang for their buck, they'll proceed to buy the largest bag available. While it's true that the larger bags are usually more economical on a per pound/kilogram basis—making it a better deal for you—it may be a bad deal for Whiskers or Spot. The issue here is freshness. Once you open the bag and introduce it to air, it begins to go stale, and eventually to spoil. There is this mistaken belief that, being dry food, it can last for an indefinite period of time. Not so!

Yes, it's dry food . . . but it's still food. The longer you have it, the staler it becomes.

I have actually refused to sell a bag of food I considered to be too large for the destined pet. Almost all customers respect my advice, but a few have walked out, not willing to listen to information that will give them a healthier pet at a daily price increase less than that they would spend—without a thought—on a cup of coffee. You aren't saving anything if your dog or cat is consuming garbage by taking too long to eat its way to the bottom of the bag. Ideally, I prefer my customers to purchase a bag size that the pet will consume in approximately four weeks. Five weeks is okay; six weeks is pushing my comfort zone. Eight weeks is, in my opinion, the maximum time in which your four-footed family member should be eating that bag of food. However, there are some factors that influence this time frame that are beyond my knowledge; I don't know what the storage conditions are in your home, or how you're storing the food (containers, etc.). Those and other factors are important when considering how long you have an opened bag of food in the home.

Tip: One way you can economize with a large bag size and still retain freshness is by freezing a portion of the food. Simply rebag some into handy plastic freezer bags and retrieve them from the freezer when needed. This also works well with canned food; divide the food into serving portions, then wrap and freeze.

Some customers are confused as to what a best before date is. That's the date the manufacturer suggests their product be sold and used by. Regardless of when you purchase the product, once you open the bag, the date is no longer applicable. Upon opening the bag, the clock commences ticking immediately as oxidation and other factors such as storage conditions now come into play to determine how long the food retains its suitability for feeding. Forgive my redundancy, as this is important . . . about four weeks is ideal for an open bag to be used up. Eight weeks is, in my opinion, the absolute maximum length I'd suggest for finishing an open bag . . . but only if stored under ideal conditions.

Here's a horror story that may keep you awake tonight. It reinforces my points made in this chapter and especially in the prior section, Storing Pet Food. Stephen King couldn't dream up anything as frightful as this.

A lady came into my store one afternoon, referred to me by one of her friends. She needed some advice regarding her dog's health. It took about thirty minutes of conversation to drag out the details of her pet's predicament. Here's her story.

About a year prior, she had adopted a small terrier cross from the local shelter. He was a neutered male weighing less than ten pounds. The problem was, for the past two or three months, the dog had been suffering from chronic diarrhea, howled at mealtimes, and vomited frequently. She had taken him to her vet on several occasions, where the poor dog had been carefully examined . . . with no cause for the problems identified. The problems continued, with the dog experiencing diarrhea just that morning. Here's the information I eventually uncovered during our conversation, some of it like pulling teeth from a chicken.

When she adopted the dog, the shelter provided her with a discount coupon for use at a local pet food store (not my store, thank heaven). Being price conscious, she had bought a forty-pound bag of dog food for her new companion. It was now about a year later, and the dog was still being fed from the same initial bag of food (not surprising considering the size of the dog). That's right, almost a year later! As terrible as that is, the story gets worse.

She and the dog lived in a small apartment. As there was no convenient place inside the apartment to keep the large bag of food, it was stored out on the apartment's exposed balcony. Yes, outside! We're in a northern climate here. That meant, for a year, this bag had been outside in summer's heat and humidity, winter's freeze and thaw cycles, and everything in between, day in, day out! If an unopened bag of food had been stored in such conditions, it would be garbage after all that time. I can't begin to imagine the disgusting condition of the food in an open bag. Now the dog was constantly sick, howling in misery each time she served up a dish of rancid, decomposing food. By the time she came to me, the remaining food was probably unfit even for maggots.

Once I finally figured this all out, I suggested she buy a small bag of fresh food immediately, even though she noted there was still almost a quarter of the original bag left. It belongs in the garbage, I advised her. Apparently this message utterly failed to sink in. No, instead of dumping it in the garbage, she thought she'd drop it off at the shelter for them to use up. I'm sorry to say that's when I yelled at her. I don't recall what I said to her, but it certainly wasn't complimentary. It's the only time in my lengthy retail career that I ever actually lost my cool with a customer.

There are a couple of issues associated with the above horror story. When new paropets come into my store, I always have a chat with them about their new family member. From that, I can determine the approximate age and size of the dog or cat and whether or not there's more than one pet in the family. That and other information assists me in determining an appropriate food . . . and bag size. Regarding the above story, apparently my competitor, a corporate chain store, had no interest beyond selling her a bag of food, the larger the better.

The second issue has to do with the several trips the woman made to the vet clinic. We'll overlook the fact that these visits must have cost her a great deal more than the money she saved in buying the largest bag size available. The ongoing vomiting and diarrhea was an instant clue for me that there might be a food issue here. Sure, it could be something else, but, with those symptoms, it's pretty much the first thing anyone should investigate. Call it a no-brainer! It bothers me greatly that any vet would fail to identify the cause of this poor dog's misery, especially after repeat visits for the same problem. With a few questions they could have solved this pet's health issue on the first visit. And they should have!

Don't buy a bag of food that is too large for your cat or dog to eat within a reasonable period of time. Any money you think you're saving on food may well end up in your veterinarian's pocket.

SWITCHING FOODS/ROTATION DIETS

If you have a glutton in the house like my dog Taffy, switching from one food to another is never a problem. Taffy will eat anything, anytime, anywhere. Actually, she doesn't so much eat her food as inhale it: we should have named her Dyson, after the vacuum cleaner. Maybe that's why her teeth have remained so clean over the years—nothing much comes in contact with them. I have learned, however, that all cats and dogs are not like Taffy when it comes to eating. Some are fussy, and this curse seems to weigh more heavily on cats than dogs. Actually, cats may be beyond fussy and are better described as persnickety. You have no idea how many times I've had desperate cat parents in my store, staring blankly at foods while wondering if their cat will eat it. For some cat owners, it can become a problem straight from hell if a manufacturer discontinues a product that was the ONLY food their cat would eat. From a cat's straightforward point of view, if it did something once it's because it was always done that way and should always be done that way. No changes without consent, thank you!

At the heart of the problem is our proclivity to feed our cats and dogs a single diet. The trend, for as long as I can remember, has always been to put our pet on a food and keep him/her on that food until the day he/she dies. Even vets have been strong supporters of that philosophy, as once was I. However, if you pause to reflect on it, it just doesn't make any sense: in fact, you could easily make a case that it defies common sense. I'm paranoid enough to suspect this nonsensical viewpoint was put into play decades ago by a pet food manufacturer intent on having you keep Spot and Whiskers on his diet, thus one-upping his competitors. That may not be true, but it makes me happy to think so.

Gradually, as I dealt more and more with allergic pets over the course of many years, I became suspicious of this established feeding practice. Eventually, I concluded that this practice of sticking with a single diet was actually detrimental to the long-term nutritional health of our pets, and furthermore, contributed significantly to fussy eater syndrome.

The reason we don't like to switch our pet's diets is simple: switching all too frequently leads to vomiting and diarrhea. The cause of this digestive problem is not difficult to understand. All animals, including humans, rely on enzymes and intestinal florae (beneficial bacteria) to assist us in digesting our food. The process commences right in our mouths when enzyme-rich saliva mixes with food during chewing. Bacteria, along with digestive enzymes and stomach acids, break down our foods into minute particles, which can be absorbed into the body as nutrients. I believe the problem of vomiting/diarrhea occurs because the pet's florae deal with the same food day after day, month after month, and rarely have an opportunity to adjust to other foods. In essence, I think the florae become lazy, or perhaps unskilled, on a single, monotonous diet. Give them something else to eat and they can't handle it. Presto . . . vomiting and diarrhea!

I never feed more than two bags in a row of the same food to Taffy. Her diet is switched frequently. I have done this same feeding regimen with my springer spaniel, Cinnamon, with the same nonresults . . . no vomiting, no diarrhea. Many of my customers are successfully following a similar feeding protocol. This type of feeding has become more widespread and is now referred to as a "rotation" diet.

Simply put, I'm of the opinion that cats and dogs should NOT be fed the same food all of the time. They should not be restricted to a single diet day in, day out, year after year. As stated above, if you take a minute to think about it, it just doesn't make any sense to feed anything that way. You wouldn't raise your children on a diet consisting of a single vitaminized cereal, would you? Changing diets regularly, I believe, will benefit your pet's health and help eliminate tendencies toward fussiness and allergies as a result of staying with a single food.

When new puppy or kitten owners come into my store to shop for an appropriate food, I always recommend not picking out only one food. Instead, I suggest they select two, preferably three, foods that meet their criteria. Each food should be from a different manufacturer in order to maximize benefits resulting from change. (The foods can be from the same manufacturer if you ensure that the meat and other major ingredients are sufficiently varied.) Feed the first food for a bag or two, then move to the second and do the same, then on to the third selection for another one or two bags, then return to the first food and repeat the process. Be sure to transition from one bag to the next by blending over a period of ten or more days.

Tip: This process can be simplified if your pet food retailer has a computerized cash system that allows them to track customer purchases. With this information, they can tell you what brand and how many you've purchased recently.

With this agenda, I can pretty much guarantee that you will not end up with a fussy eater who'll freak out at the sight of anything new in its dish. Further, I firmly believe your pet will have fewer health issues over the coming years. Also, transitioning your cat or dog from one diet to another, if done frequently as I recommend, will not likely create the problem of vomiting or diarrhea. The more frequently you change your pet's food, the more readily change will be accepted by their digestive partners. You and I eat a wide variety of foodstuffs daily without suffering from intestinal problems because our intestinal florae have adapted to variety. Once the pet's florae become accustomed to an assortment of various products, incidents of vomiting or diarrhea relating to a change in food should vanish.

That's well and good for kittens and puppies. Like most children, they're curious and accepting. It's usually quite easy to implement the above feeding protocol with youngsters. It's a different story with adults, though; particularly with adults who have years of bad eating habits under their pelts. The problem commences when you decide to change your adult pet's diet, usually for reasons involving food quality or health issues. "Fine!" says your pet. "Let the war begin. I'm up for it. I can outsmart a two-foot any day of the week. Who do you think really calls the shots around here, pal?" From my side of the counter, it appears the four-foots are usually the ones calling the shots.

If your dog or cat has been on one food for any length of time and has a tendency toward fussiness or resistance to change, and you wish to put it on another diet, I would suggest you first approach your pet food retailer and ask for samples of other foods. You need two or three samples. Take the packages home and do your test this way: open each package and take out a small amount of the kibble. Make two or three piles about a foot from each other. Introduce your pet to the food display and see if it makes a decision. If they select and eat one of the offerings, great! End of conversation! That's the food to go with.

I had a startling demonstration of this process a few years back. A woman came in one day, worried because her Australian shepherd had stopped eating about a week earlier, following the sudden death of her husband, who the dog was very attached to. After a brief conversation, I provided her with three sample packages to take home. Instead, she left the packages on the counter and went out to her car, returning moments later with the dog. She opened each package and set the food out on the floor in the three piles, as I'd instructed. We should have videoed what followed. The Aussie carefully sniffed at each pile, one after the other. Then it returned to the first pile, sniffed again, and then sniffed the second pile. Returning to the first pile, he selected and ate a couple of pieces of kibble. He then ate a bit of food from the second pile. The third pile was now totally ignored, obviously failing to make the cut in the first round. He again favored the two preferred offerings with a sniff, followed by a quick glance at his amazed audience. Finally, decision made, he devoured everything in the first pile. His fast was over; that's the bag that went home with him.

Okay, your cat or dog has shown a preference for one of the new foods from the samples provided. When you head back to the store to buy a bag of food, do the retailer a favor . . . remember which food it was your pet selected. While that sounds silly, I can't begin to tell you how many times a customer has shown up in the store to buy a new bag of food, expecting me to know which diet their pet selected from the samples. Please, write down the name or, even better, bring along the empty packaging from the favored sample. It'll save you another trip or another round of sampling (and help prevent me from banging my head against a brick wall).

A major problem occurs when attempting to switch a cat or dog from a flavor-enhanced food to one of higher quality lacking obvious flavor enhancers such as animal digest. Remember my remark earlier about pizza diets? These, if you recall, are heavily grain-based foods generously doctored with flavor enhancers to encourage our pets to eat them. Well, a side effect of such foods is that, due to the big taste hit they provide, they end up being rather addictive (could this be an accidental side effect . . . or deliberate?). Now you wish to feed a better-quality diet—a diet that focuses on honest nutrition rather than insidious taste gimmicks. There's an excellent chance, with the first bowl of new food served, that your pet will look at you like you're totally insane. If they could, they might call an ambulance for you . . . or even the cops if they're sufficiently annoyed by your thoughtless arrogance. It's much the same reaction you'd expect from teenagers who've been surviving on cheeseburgers and pizza and now, for the first time in three years, they're facing a plate full of mashed potatoes, broccoli, unadorned chicken breast, and a salad of mixed greens. Never mind where's the meat? Where the hell is the flavor?

I have always found the greatest challenge comes from attempting to switch a pet from a flavor-enhanced diet to a quality diet. But I have my tricks, too! First, see if your pet will take a few pieces of the new kibble as treats. Often, a treat will be more acceptable than if the same thing is introduced as food. It's worth a try! If it works, keep it up for a day or two. Next, blend the new food in with the old. In addition to providing your pet's digestive system an opportunity to comfortably adjust to the new food, your cat or dog will have an opportunity to slowly adapt to the new food's scent and taste. If we're dealing with a supersensitive pet, start with adding only a few pieces of the new kibble in with the old. If that works, keep on increasing the ratio of new to old. I like a 10 percent rule. This rule says that 10 percent of the meal will consist of the new diet added to 90 percent of the old diet for the first two days, 20 percent on days three and four, 30 percent on days five and six, and so on. By the end of twenty days your pet should be eating 100 percent of the new diet. There's a reason patience is a virtue.

If you're still getting resistance to eating the new food, try adding your own flavor enhancers. My favorites are things most of us already have in the kitchen. As mentioned, dogs are a bit easier to work with than our felines; they'll be taste attracted to a wider range of flavorful things than will a cat. So for dogs, your go-to enticements (also called bribes) will be ketchup, barbeque sauce, peanut butter, beef or chicken broth, and yogurt (plain or fruit). Dogs love those big flavors, and those items will generously punch up the taste of the new food. You don't need much, usually a teaspoon or so, depending on the size of the dog. Mix the flavoring with the food and serve. None of them should be detrimental to your dog's health in the small amount you'll be applying. If that approach motivates the dog into eating the food, keep it up for two or three days, then slowly begin weaning the dog off the flavor enhancer. Also, sometimes, for some dogs, a sprinkle of garlic powder will work. Most dogs love garlic's pungent aroma; the small amount provided here will not harm their health.

If it's a frozen baked or raw diet you're trying to encourage your dog to eat, try warming up the food in the microwave for a few seconds to bring it up to room temperature. Sometimes, lightly cooking the food will help Whiskers or Spot get over the hurdle of eating raw meat. If it will eat the meal lightly cooked, slowly reduce the cooking time over several days until the food is accepted in raw condition. All of the household flavor enhancers listed in the above paragraph will work here.

Cats, as implied, are a greater challenge, mostly due to the fact that there is a much shorter list of enticements they will respond to. Yogurt, sour cream, and beef or chicken broth often get the job done. Also, mixing in a bit of canned food with the dry may do the trick. Be careful the cat doesn't just lick off the wet food and leave the remainder for the garbage can.

Remember, there's this theory out there that we humans are supposed to be smarter than cats and dogs . . . and horses and goats and so on. It's a nice thought but one that's increasingly difficult for us to substantiate. I'm confident we're smarter than grasshoppers . . . but after that, well, what can I say? I'm absolutely positive Taffy understands me much better than I understand her. Anyway, the point I wish to make here is that you, as a human, have one other option in your bag of tricks for getting your pet to eat a new food. Drum roll here, please.

Stubbornness! That's it: your hole card. Show a little determination. I can't tell you how many times a customer has come in and advised me that they put the new food down for their pet and had to throw it out an hour later because it was still in the dish. (Mind you, if it's raw food you pretty much have to throw it out before contamination sets in.) Other than raw or baked, let it sit there for an hour. It won't hurt them to miss a meal or two. As long as they have plenty of fresh water, they'll be fine for a while without food. I'd only extend this option to about three meals, and if that fails to generate the desired results, go to Plan B if you have one.

The problem with most pet owners is that we too readily succumb to The Look. That's when our adorable Whiskers or loveable Spot gazes into our eyes and a beseeching, hurtful look passes from them to us. "Please," The Look says. "Feed me my old food, even if it is full of junk ingredients." Don't be conned by The Look. It's the very same look they'll give you when attempting to mooch your meal from you.

COMPARING WET TO DRY FOODS

While the question doesn't come up often in the store, from time to time a customer will be confused by the startling difference between the values provided by the product's guaranteed analysis for a dry food and its equivalent in a canned food, per the following examples:

	Dry Food	Canned Food
Protein	22%	8%
Fat	12%	5%

If it's basically the same food, customers wonder, why are the values so disparate? The answer is, in a word, water. As mentioned earlier, the moisture content in a bag of dry food is approximately 10 percent, meaning that 10 percent of the bag's content is water and the remaining 90 percent is dry matter. Canned food, on the other hand, is mostly water, often in the 80 percent range with the remaining 20 percent being dry matter. The actual values for the moisture (water) content for both will be provided in the guaranteed analysis (perhaps the only worthwhile information in the GA).

So, in viewing the two sets of values, you are looking at an apples-to-oranges comparison; they don't match up. To turn it into a meaningful apples-to-apples comparison will require a simple math exercise. Assuming the moisture content in our bag of food is 10 percent, or 90 percent dry matter, we divide the above protein value of 22 percent by dry matter value: 22 / 90 = 24.4 percent.

Therefore, 24.4 percent is the amount of protein in the dry food calculated on a dry-matter basis.

For convenience, we are going to assume that the canned food is 80 percent water and thus 20 percent dry matter and perform a similar calculation with the 8 percent protein from the canned food above: 8 / 20 = 40 percent.

Therefore, 40 percent is the amount of protein in the canned food calculated on a dry-matter basis.

Now you have your apples-to-apples comparison. In conclusion, it's obvious that the canned food at 40 percent contains more protein per pound on a dry-matter basis than does the dry food at 24.4 percent. That's for comparative purposes only and should not be used as a part of your feeding guide. The feeding instructions on the can or bag should be your guide.

The same calculations can be used in converting all of the other guaranteed analysis values shown on both the dry food bags and canned food labels. Grab your calculator; your homework is to calculate the comparisons provided for the fat shown above.

FEEDING RULES AND REGULATIONS

One of my most frequent paropet problems involves how they are feeding their pet. It's purely a paropet problem as I can't honestly hold the pet accountable here. The issue gains in magnitude when the veterinarian insists the paropet control what and how much their pet eats. Often, these vet instructions are provided in relation to a health issue such as obesity or diabetes. After years of bad feeding habits, attempting to change an established feeding regimen can turn a pet-happy home into a war zone. Why a war zone? Well, dogs and cats don't like change; even more so than we two-foots, they are creatures of habit.

The biggest feeding mistake perpetrated by well-meaning but thoughtless pet parents is free-feeding. Free-feeding is when there's unlimited food constantly in the bowl and the cat or dog is allowed to eat whenever it's in a mood to do so, whether hungry or bored. How, when, and why did this become a good idea? There are only two times when I can approve of free-feeding: when you have a very young kitten or puppy, or when caring for a pregnant bitch or queen (more on pregnancy/nursing shortly). For the youngsters, because they're so active and growing so fast, free-feeding is a good idea—but only for a few weeks. Once they've reached approximately three months of age, no more free-feeding. From three to six months, puppies and kittens should receive three meals daily. After six months, they should receive two meals a day.

I am aware that some pets actually do quite well free-feeding. It appears they have self-control and don't turn into hogs at the trough. Taffy would not be one of these. If I allowed her to free-feed, I'd have to hire someone to fill her food dish all day long. She'd go from thirty pounds to three hundred pounds in no time at all. Still, even for those pets who demonstrate greater responsibility than their owners, free-feeding is a bad idea. Situations can change over time. A cat that has been responsible for its own eating habits can, in later years, become less active or develop other health issues, and the feeding protocol may be a factor. If it continues eating the same amount of food daily, eventually it will start to gain unwanted weight.

Warning: A serious downside to free-feeding is the practice's relationship to disease. As well as a tendency toward obesity, animals allowed to free-feed are also more prone to heart disease, some forms of arthritis, and diabetes.

The following advice involves those of you free-feeding kibble: if you're feeding raw, baked, or canned food, you should not be allowing those meals to remain in the dish for more than thirty minutes . . . ever.

It's time for some tough love if you wish to introduce controlled feeding. In order to prevent a situation in which your house is turned into an unpleasant combat zone, here's my suggestion for weaning your cat or dog off its free-feeding joyride. For homes in which a two-foot is present all day, implementation is relatively easy. Commencing about midday, remove the food dish for an hour or two. Do that for two or three days. Objections should be minimal, if any. Then expand on the "no food" period by extending the time for an hour on each end (remove the food an hour earlier and replace it an hour later), and continue this for an additional two or three days. Keep expanding the "no food" period outward from the middle: eventually food will only be available for an hour in the morning and another hour in the evening. The one point to keep in mind here is to not attempt this change quickly. Two or more weeks would be ideal. The slower you implement the new regimen, the more acceptable it will be to your pet and the less likely to create confrontation.

Once you have the food down for an hour in the morning and another in the evening, the final step is to reduce the "food available" time to about thirty minutes for each period. Any food not eaten in the half hour should be discarded, and don't forget to wash out the food dish after each meal. For homes where humans are absent most of the day, it can be more challenging implementing a feeding change. Is there a trusted friend or neighbor who can help? If yes, then they can help you to implement the above plan. If not, you may have to go cold turkey. Put out the pet's food as soon as you get up in the morning and remove it just prior to leaving the house. As soon as someone arrives home in the evening, put food down, allowing food to be available for an hour or more with each meal. Continue to shorten the length of time the food is available until eventually, food is only presented for that thirty-minute period twice daily.

PREGNANCY AND NURSING

It is difficult to imagine a time when good nutrition is more important than during a mother's pregnancy and nursing period. For the mother, adequate nutrition is not good enough; she requires the best food available both for herself and for the kittens or puppies coming into the world. If you have been scrimping on your pet food budget for whatever reason, now is the time to reconsider, as good nutrition should be the priority throughout this period.

There is an exception to every rule, and the exception to not free-feeding adults comes into play when dealing with pregnant or nursing pets. However, free-feeding here does not imply unlimited quantity. The package's feeding instructions for pregnant/lactating females should be your guide. These instructions usually recommend an increase in food that might be better presented as frequent smaller meals instead of one or two large meals.

Pregnancy and birth is a very stressful time for any mother. In fact, it can be so stressful that many bitches will "blow their coat," an event were they lose a great deal of their hair within a few days. Nutrition's role in dealing with stress cannot be understated. I recall a breeder of huskies in a nearby community who, a few years ago, decided to see for herself if food would make a difference with two bitches that were about to deliver their pups only about one week apart. Early in their pregnancies, we discussed a suitable diet, with the second dog (Dog B) being put on the new food, one of significantly improved quality in comparison to that which all of her other dogs were receiving, including the other pregnant dog (Dog A). Dog B was gently weaned onto her new diet during the first two weeks of her pregnancy.

Following birth, both of the new mothers blew their coats as anticipated. The breeder did notice that Dog B, on the superior diet, suffered less hair loss than did Dog A. Further, even though Dog B birthed her litter about a week later than Dog A, her coat returned to its full glory much faster than that of Dog A. While not a clinical test, the breeder was suitably impressed with the obvious benefits of feeding a high-quality food, so much so that all of her dogs began enjoying a better diet following that feeding trial.

A good quality All Life Stages food is satisfactory for a pregnant or nursing mother. If you're using a food that has a puppy or kitten formula available, then you should begin feeding that formula as it will provide the much-needed additional nutrition to mom and her babies. If a change in the food is in order, I prefer to make the switch as early in the pregnancy as possible, when the change will create the least amount of additional stress on the mother. In fact, if this is a planned pregnancy, I would recommend the diet be switched prior to the fertilization event.

Pregnant cats and dogs can go through a brief period of appetite loss, similar to morning sickness. Usually, this will pass in about a week. Other than that, you should expect to have the mother gradually increase the amount of food she eats on a daily basis. For this period I suggest controlled free-feeding the mother as this is not a good time to ration her nutrition. (This is about the only time when controlled free-feeding an adult pet is the sensible thing to do.) Continue the free-feeding routine throughout both the pregnancy and nursing periods, and for at least one month after the pups or kittens have been weaned (unless she starts putting on unwanted weight). After that, transition her back to a normal twice-daily feeding routine. If your pregnant cat or dog has a tendency toward gluttony at the best of times, to the point where free-feeding may prove to be a negative rather than a positive, you can consider providing a series of small meals rather than keeping the bowl full of food—just be sure that you provide sufficient food for mother and babies.

Note: It is extremely important to ensure that the pregnant or nursing mother has an ample supply of fresh water available to her at all times. This is even more important for cats and smaller dogs, which, due to their smaller body mass, can become dehydrated more rapidly than larger pets.

Moderate exercise is still important for pregnant and nursing mothers. If other pets are in the family, she should be protected from any roughhousing or other strenuous play they may customarily indulge in. Cats normally allowed to roam should be kept indoors, especially during the last two or three weeks of their pregnancy, and while still nursing. I don't believe cats should be allowed to roam at any time. If you can convince her to remain indoors for this period, why not just keep her indoors in the future now that she's adjusted to being confined?

During the pregnancy and nursing period, it is vitally important to ensure your veterinarian is involved in monitoring the mother's health during the process. Your vet may likely do a thorough physical exam and will be the source of good advice on how to prepare for the pending increase in your family's size. If you even suspect your cat or dog is pregnant, your vet must be made aware of this, as no vaccinations should be administered at this time.

Will good nutrition provided to a mother benefit her pups or kittens? In the chapter on osteoarthritis I state, "There is also a suspicion that generational factors working in combination may lead to the onset of the disease (specifically, generations of dogs on poor-quality diets combined with generations of poor breeding practices may be, and likely are, major contributors to the problem)." A mother on a nutritious diet will deliver stronger, healthier babies; these fortunate puppies and kittens will enjoy better health later in their own lives, compliments of their mother's nutritional health.

Good nutrition is a win-win for everyone . . . every time.

Another feeding problem I often face when dealing with customers is determining exactly how much food is ending up in the pet's dish. You'd be astounded to learn how many people really don't know how much food they're serving Whiskers or Spot with each meal. Are you one of these guilty people? They think they know how much they're serving, but they really don't have a clue. These paropets use something to scoop—or just pour out—what they consider to be an appropriate amount of food, either canned or kibble. If there's more than one person involved in feeding the cat or dog, then there are two or more versions of what's a sufficient serving. If that's what you're doing, you are looking for trouble.

Use a measuring cup! That's all it takes. They aren't expensive. Know how much food is appropriate for your companion and serve a proper, measured meal. How can it be any easier than that? Ensure that everyone involved in feeding the four-foots knows exactly how much is to be served with each meal. In this way, should your pet lose or gain too much weight, you can increase/decrease the amount of food you're providing in a sensible, controlled manner.

Life becomes complicated in multipet, free-feeding households when one pet decides the food in the other guy's dish tastes better than the food in its own dish, or is just a glutton and gobbles down its own food before rushing to help empty the other bowl(s) in the house. In that scenario we often end up with one overweight and one underweight pet. Now you're forced to introduce feeding controls to two or more cats and/or dogs. It won't be fun. The only way to solve this issue is to make the food available for about thirty minutes and ensure both pets cannot access each other's meal. This may entail feeding them in separate rooms or implementing other restrictions. In cat/dog scenarios, it's usually the dog trying to steal the cat's food. Often, placing the cat's dish in a high location, accessible only to the cat, will solve this problem.

When do you switch your pets from kitten or puppy formulas to adult formulas? This is another frequently asked question. It's a question with no firm answer because it has more to do with basic common sense than with a date on a calendar. Opinions are so varied on this topic that if you ask eight people you'll likely end up with ten answers.

The most rapid growth period for kittens and puppies is the first six months. After that, growth and energy requirements start slowing as they continue maturing. Some cats can reach maturity at about nine months, smaller dogs at around one year, with giant breeds maturing at up to two years. Generally speaking, you should consider switching your cat to adult food at six or seven months and small breed dogs at around one year. For medium and large dog breeds, six to nine months of age is suitable. For giant breeds, switch to adult food at about four or five months.

As a guideline, the above is a generalization only. For example, many people dislike putting large and giant breeds on a puppy formula in the first place, as they wish to discourage rapid growth, a potential cause of health problems later in life. Instead, their big puppy is weaned directly onto an adult food. This is fine as long as the quality of the food is sufficient for good nutrition. In this situation, an All Life Stages food is likely superior to a standard adult food. Foods with excessive calorie and calcium content should be avoided for large breed puppies.

You can avoid the whole scenario if you're wise enough to use a good-quality All Life Stages product for your puppy or kitten. Rather than switching, you simply need to monitor how much food you're feeding your puppy or kitten. Older animals that have completed, or nearly completed, their growth require less food than younger, growing pets. Refer to the feeding guideline on the package, keeping in mind it is only a guide. You must also consider the genetic heritage of your pet. Cats such as Siamese and dogs such as greyhounds and whippets are at their best when on the lean side: if a pug is thin, it needs more food; if a whippet is thin, it's fine.

The common sense I mentioned comes into play throughout your pet's lifetime from youngster to adult to senior. Monitor your pet's weight at all times. Spot's and Whiskers's actual weight should dictate what and how much is being fed more so than a date on a calendar or advice on a package. A kitten or puppy that's too thin should probably remain on puppy or kitten food for a while longer, or, if using an All Life Stages formula, continue feeding a larger food amount until their weight comes into line with expectations. If the pet becomes too chubby, then consider moving them to an adult formula, or reducing the amount of All Life Stages being fed.

Again, let common sense be your guide.

Another feeding issue customers ask about from time to time involves feeding a combination of canned food (wet) and kibble (dry). Is it okay to do so? I'm not sure this question ever came up prior to the arrival of raw diets into the pet world. There's a belief in the "raw" community that you cannot mix raw with kibble as the two are digested at different rates and processed through the gut at different speeds, and serious gastrointestinal problems will result from mixing the two. Having fed raw/kibble combinations to my dogs, if there's any truth at all in this view, my dogs' intestines failed to recognize it.

So, yes, you can mix wet and dry food, or raw and dry. Some customers feed wet food for one meal and dry food for the next. Others blend a bit of both at each meal, leading to the question of how much of each should be provided. You can do a lot of calculating in trying to figure this out, but my simple rule of thumb is to serve, in combination, the amount of food that would constitute one meal. This means if Spot is supposed to receive one cup of kibble at each feeding, and now you wish to add in some canned food, then you will serve one cup of a combination of canned and dry foods. Scientifically correct, no; it will do until you can afford to hire a pet nutritionist.

To ensure that's sufficient food, simply monitor Whiskers's or Spot's weight from time to time (which you should be doing anyway). If their weight drops, increase their food; if weight increases, reduce the combined amount of food until their weight returns to a suitable level.

DAVE'S TABLE SCRAP RULES

Another frequent topic of conversation with pet parents is that of feeding table scraps. As I make my living by selling pet food, it may come as a surprise to some of you to discover I have no problem with feeding leftovers. Sure it cuts into my profits, but it's all about our pets, not me.

I didn't realize that feeding leftovers was controversial until I attended a seminar some years back conducted by a well-known pet nutritionist who consults with pet food manufacturers around the world. He was adamant in his opinion that table scraps should never be provided to pets. NEVER! In his opinion, additional foodstuffs will throw off the delicate balance of vitamins and minerals that are carefully and professionally crafted into each and every bite of pet food. Even today, when I wander about the Internet, I find the same cautions being provided for the same reasons. Frankly, I feel bad for any pet living with that consultant: what a drab dietary life that poor creature must lead. Considering that our pets have survived and thrived by mooching off us for centuries, I failed to buy into his philosophy then and still don't to this day.

I think leftovers can be beneficial to our pets' diets nutritionally, and as well, put a smile on their furry faces. However, when it comes to feeding table leftovers, I do have some rules. You may want to copy these rules out and post them where Whiskers, Spot, and the rest of your family (especially husbands) can read them. I identify husbands as a problem here because, based on my years of experience, when it comes to sneaking food to a pet, husbands are at the top of the list of guilty perpetrators, followed by children. Sorry, guys, but I know that you know this is true.

Rule #1:   Leftovers designated for your pet should consist of lean meat and vegetables. The skin from the chicken or the wedge of fat from the roast that you consider unfit for you is also unfit for your pet to eat. Skin and fat aren't leftovers; they're garbage. Be sure to remove any small bones from poultry and fish.

Rule #2:   All things in moderation. A small amount of leftovers will make your pet smile. Too much and you may trigger the vomiting/diarrhea problem mentioned earlier. Also, the more frequently your pet receives some leftovers, the less likely it will experience those gastro-intestinal problems. If you have too much food left over, split up your pet's leftover servings into smaller portions and serve over successive meals.

Note: The frequent provision of leftovers may instill the expectation of leftovers with some pets. They may then refuse to eat their regular diet if it isn't adorned with something special. Do not cater to picky eaters. Leftovers are best served as an occasional mealtime treat. Make them a pleasant surprise rather than an entitlement.

Rule #3:   Portion control is important. I rarely serve more than half a meal of leftovers, with the remaining half consisting of their regular diet. The total amount of food served when leftovers are included will not exceed a normal serving of their regular food. If you unthinkingly provide a regular meal and then add some leftovers, you're on your way to an obese pet.

Rule #4:   To prevent mooching you need to separate your meal from the serving of leftovers. Your goal is to eliminate any association between your plate and the pet's bowl, so leftovers do not go directly from plate to bowl. Instead, refrigerate any leftovers designated for your four-foot and include them with one of its meals the following day.

Rule #5:   Fruit and veggie snacks. Your cat won't likely care, but your dog is usually interested in sharing these snacks with you. Taffy, for instance, would stand on her head (if she could) for a piece of carrot. A slice of your apple or peach or a bit of banana or other fruit, and most vegetables, make a great addition to your pet's diet. The advice in Rule #2 remains applicable: all things in moderation.

Rule #6:   Leftovers are not recommended for young puppies and kittens under six months old. Rule #2 is very important for this group.

Warning: Grapes, raisins, and onions should NOT be given to your pet at any time, on their own or mixed with other foods. All are toxic.

PET FOOD MYTHS

I'm always astounded by the number of myths floating around regarding pet foods. Many years ago I worked in the wine industry and assumed, when it came to food myths, that wine was impossible to beat. I still think wine myths outnumber those of pet foods, but I'm surprised at how many this industry possesses. We've covered most of these points earlier, but the following is provided as an easily remembered summary.

If it's shown on TV it must be good.

Yeah, sure! While some quality diets are now being advertised on television and in print media, their appearance is a recent event. For most of the years I've been in the pet food business, I have never seen an advertisement for a food I considered suitable for any of my pets. The bottom line for most advertised foods is this: the money either goes into quality ingredients or into shareholder's pockets. Lots of inexpensive grain and undesirable protein sources in the diet supports heavy advertising and shareholders. Don't be duped by slick commercials. Also, I'm always suspicious if they use veterinarians for touting the food as, like actors, they're probably well compensated for their endorsements.

Dry pet food stays good forever.

Come on now! It's food! Heat, moisture, and contact with air will eventually cause the food to lose its freshness, degrade its nutrition, and finally cause it to turn rancid and then decompose. Only buy a bag size that your cat or dog can use up quickly, ideally within four to six weeks.

Is there any difference between a holistic, premium, super premium or ultra premium food?

The question is irrelevant as there are no regulations covering the use of those words for describing a pet food. The terms are without value, or, harshly put, they are meaningless. These adjectives can be applied to the worst pet food in the world.

It's OK to store dog food in other containers.

Big no-no! If the other container is a food-grade container, then fine. The best thing to do is to leave the food in its original package, wipe down the storage container with a disinfectant, and store the food and package in the other container. Keep as much air as possible away from the food. Do not use any container not designed for food storage, especially if it's made of plastic.

It's OK to let pets free-feed (food is always in the dish).

It's okay for young kittens and puppies, as well as pregnant and nursing mothers, but not for too long. Eventually, you want to reduce the free-feeding to three meals daily. By about three months, puppies and kittens should be down to two meals daily, and lactating mothers the same shortly after weaning, with the food left out for about thirty minutes tops.

Pet foods are complete diets because of the supporting research.

There's been more research on human diets than for any other animal on earth and we still don't know how to feed ourselves properly. If we did, obesity wouldn't be a problem of epidemic proportion worldwide. AAFCO's pet feeding trials need only last twenty-six weeks, with questionable controls in place during that period. These controls seem to favor the manufacturer more than our cats and dogs.

You should never change your pet's diet.

Why not? This myth has been around for decades. I suspect it was started by clever pet food manufacturers as it has all of the appearances of being one of those self-serving statements. Changing diets from time to time will contribute to a healthier pet over the years.

Table scraps are bad for pets.

Says who? Don't try to sell that one to Taffy. It's another myth that's survived for decades and should be relegated to a myth trash heap. Good-quality leftovers will put a smile on your pet's face. Just keep in mind my rules for feeding leftovers.

Dry pet food helps keep teeth clean.

I've never seen any proof of this in spite of the fact many pet owners seem to accept it as gospel. Most cats and dogs having their teeth cleaned at their vet's office were eating dry kibble in part or whole. Personally, I believe starchy diets are a major contributor to a pet's dental problems. Quality diets that are not starchy appear to provide a superior oral benefit for our four-foots.

WHAT'S MISSING?

We mentioned the AAFCO feeding trials earlier. There is one feeding trial conducted by manufacturers, the results of which don't appear on their packaging. You're lucky! I'm talking about palatability trials. How tasty is the food? Every company representative that's come into my store promoting their terrific new pet food has quickly mentioned the superior palatability it possesses. They do feeding trials with the new diet using competitor's foods as the standard by which they measure their own food. We never know what competitor foods are used

(I've asked reps and they had no idea). All they know is that their food proved far more acceptable to the cats/dogs involved in the taste tests than any other of the competitive diets. Further, as standards for palatability trials may be nonexistent, the whole concept may be no more than a bad joke on consumers.

Of course their diet proved superior in palatability. Duh! Can you imagine a salesperson walking into a pet food retailer and saying, "Hey, I've got this terrific new food I'd like you to carry in your store. It has great quality and is very healthy. The downside is that cats and dogs think it tastes worse than sun-dried lizard poop, and they refuse to eat it."

That'll never happen! No, every food that's ever been introduced to me has been more palatable than any other food that's gone before it. Yeah, sure! I, of course, have no way of determining how acceptable any new diet is to a pet. I can only take their word for it. But I'm a skeptic! In order for both my customers and I to be protected from these unsupportable claims, I have a single recourse. If they think most dogs and cats will eat this food, I insist they put their money where their mouth is. If my customers' pets refuse to eat it, will they take the uneaten food back and authorize a full credit for my customer? They need to say "yes"' to that question.

They really don't have much of a choice if they want stores like mine to list the product for sale. Really, it's a win-win-win for everyone. As manufacturers, they get their products into the consumer's home. If they've done their job right, most pets will eat the food: win some, lose some. As a retailer, I can promote a new food, assured that I can make things right for any unsatisfied customer whose pet rejects the food. The paropet has the privilege of trying a new food with Whiskers or Spot, knowing that any rejection by the pet will not be money wasted.

Tip: If you're test-driving a new diet with your pet, before putting your money down, inquire as to the retailer's return policy in the event the food is refused. This advice covers pet food retailers as well as veterinarian clinics that sell pet food.

LESSONS LEARNED

The purpose behind most of the preceding chapters was to teach you how to become an informed consumer when shopping for your pet's food, and how to manage the provision of food. As pointed out early on, if you're not an informed consumer then you'll likely be an uninformed dupe, a victim of clever marketing tactics or misleading information provided by the Internet and misguided acquaintances. You may be cheated at the cash register by paying too much for a food that provides too little, and Spot or Whiskers may be cheated nutritionally. You may even become a victim of your pet's manipulations, as we've just finished discussing. Before moving on to other topics, the following points summarize what you've learned so far:

- You no longer have any excuse for feeding your dog or cat a poor-quality diet.
- You know what information is of greatest value to you on the package, and how to understand that information.
- You know how to determine good ingredients from bad and recognize ingredients that may be included for the sole purpose of impressing you rather than providing a nutritional benefit to Whiskers or Spot. When reviewing ingredients always question their suitability for a carnivore.
- Misleading terms such as *holistic*, *ultra*, *super*, or *premium*, alone or in combination, will no longer deceive you.
- You will not believe the first thing you read about pet diets on the Internet. Instead, you will investigate other sources to determine the creditability of the information. Those sources can be pet food suppliers, trainers, breeders, library, and Internet sites.
- You are highly suspicious of misleading or generic wording.
- You view manufacturer's websites, advertisements, and commercials with righteous skepticism. (These websites can contain valuable information; you are responsible for determining that which is valuable from that which is propaganda.)
- You will apply that same skepticism toward the many pet food blogs found online.

You are now an informed consumer. Congratulations!

CHAPTER 5

It's Hard to Beat a Good Treat

No matter how much cats fight, there always seem to be plenty of kittens.

—Abraham Lincoln

No food-related conversation is complete without a discussion on pet treats, as treats are also food. We all love food treats. For me, chocolate will do it every time. I suspect that, in its own way, just about every mammal, bird, and fish has a favorite food, something they consider to be a treat. Our favorite food may not be the healthiest thing for us to eat: regardless, it's our favorite food . . . and that's what counts.

For most people in the business of training animals, food rewards are the preferred method for capturing the interest of a creature that otherwise demonstrates an attention deficit disorder. It isn't that they actually suffer from attention deficit; it's just that they aren't too interested in learning the things we want them to know. That's where treats come in. The more food driven a pet is, the easier it is to train them. The only other requirements are patience and a reasonable level of intelligence in both the trainer and trainee (it only becomes embarrassing when the trainee is smarter than the trainer).

I have customers who agonize over the selection of their pets' treats as much as they do over what food to feed them. That's fine! They obviously care about their cat or dog, and that's always a good thing. When asked for my advice, I will question them about a few things such as the pet's age, preferences, and allergy concerns. Once I acquire some basic information, we can discuss an appropriate treat for Whiskers or Spot.

You've probably assumed by now that I'm not a fan of junk treats. While I do carry a limited selection of them, I never recommend them to customers. What I'm referring to here as a junk treat is, in my opinion, those soft, chewy, moist treats containing undesirable ingredients such as by-products and dyes. Their popularity results from mass-market merchandising supported by frequent advertising campaigns (those like Super Cat smashing through a wall in search of a treat). My dogs have never had as much as a single bite of any of these treats, and I consider them the better for it. They're popular with cats and dogs because they provide a huge taste hit thanks to all of the salt, sugar, and other flavorings added for palatability. They also add other undesirable ingredients such as mystery meats, by-products, dyes, chemical preservatives such as ethoxyquin and BHT, and enough other chemicals to impress a chemist. Here's the ingredient list from one popular mass-market dog treat: ground wheat, corn gluten meal, wheat flour, ground yellow corn, water, sugar, glycerin, soybean meal, hydrogenated starch hydrolysate, bacon (preserved with sodium nitrite), salt, bacon fat (preserved with BHA), meat, phosphoric acid, sorbic acid (a preservative), dried cheese powder, calcium propionate (a preservative), natural and artificial smoke flavors, added color (red 40, yellow 6, blue 1).

There are lots of things to dislike here—all of it, in fact. In the first four ingredients, two are wheat and two are corn products; all are associated with causing allergies, as is the soybean meal further along. Sugar and salt are supplied in generous portions. Glycerin adds more sweetness and helps the product retain moisture for the soft/chewy texture. Nitrites and BHA as preservatives have been dropped by most pet food manufacturers but are included here. A mystery meat is used. Three dyes are provided for your visual benefit, not your dog's health.

It's no better for felines. Here's an ingredient list from a popular mass-market cat treat: chicken by-product meal, ground corn, animal fat (preserved with mixed tocopherols), rice, dried meat by-products, wheat flour, natural flavors, corn gluten meal, tapioca starch, minerals (potassium chloride, zinc sulphate, calcium carbonate, iron oxide, copper sulfate, manganese sulfate, potassium iodide), cellulose, sodium tripolyphosphate, vitamins (choline chloride, l-ascorbyl-2-polyphosphate [source of vitamin C*], folic acid, dl-alpha tocopherol acetate [source of vitamin E], vitamin A supplement, niacin supplement, vitamin B12 supplement, riboflavin supplement, thiamine mononitrate [vitamin B1], D-calcium pantothenate, vitamin D3 supplement, biotin, pyridoxine hydrochloride [vitamin B6], sodium carboxy methyl cellulose, salt, taurine, dl-methionine, green tea extract.

There are lots of things to toss darts at with this cat treat: by-product meat meal, mystery animal fat and meat, wheat, corn fractions, cellulose, and unidentified (natural?) flavors. The long supplement cocktail is about the only good news here; I suppose we should be grateful for the vitamins they've added as none were provided for Spot in the above dog product.

I won't go into greater detail here as most of the items I dislike have been discussed in chapter 2, but now you know why I don't recommend these types of treats and refuse to feed them, even in small amounts, to my pets. Regrettably, these types of treat products dominate retailers' shelves in pet food stores, supermarkets, and convenience stores. And don't forget, many of those questionable ingredients are approved by AAFCO.

If it's a soft, chewy treat you're interested in, then there are some better options available in many pet food supply outlets. In chapter 2 I tried to reinforce the idea of reading the package ingredient list. My advice for treats remains the same: if you want a chewy treat with quality ingredients, start by reading the list of ingredients. Here, in comparison to the above ingredient lists, is a soft, chewy treat I would feed to Taffy: chicken, venison, ground brown rice, oatmeal, vegetable glycerin, guar gum, cane molasses, carrots, salt, natural smoke flavor, garlic, blueberries, flaxseed, sweet potatoes, apples, phosphoric acid (a natural acidifier), sorbic acid (a preservative), and mixed tocopherols (a natural preservative).

There's little in the above list to offend a concerned paropet. All of the ingredients appear to be superior in quality when compared to the two preceding dog and cat treats. Included are two whole grains that follow—rather than lead the two meats. Two vegetables and two fruits are provided, possibly to impress the buyer more than to benefit the user. I'd prefer not to have any sweetener, such as molasses, as the berries, apples, and sweet potatoes should adequately fill this need.

Will healthier treats be more expensive than the other products shown? Yes, they will. Quality usually (but not always) costs more. The healthier option could be twice the price of the other two versions. In my opinion, the extra money is still worth it for your peace of mind, especially when you consider that these are treats, not a main diet. As treats, you should only be doling these items out in small amounts on occasion, not as a major part of your pet's daily food intake.

It's a similar story when it comes to selecting dog biscuits. There are countless varieties available. When it comes to quality, however, all are not equal. Here's the ingredient list from a popular, widely distributed brand: wheat flour, wheat bran, meat and bone meal, milk, wheat germ, beef fat (preserved with tocopherols), salt, natural flavor, dicalcium phosphate, calcium carbonate, brewer's dried yeast, malted barley flour, sodium metabisulfite (used as a preservative), choline chloride, minerals (ferrous sulfate, zinc oxide, manganous oxide, copper sulfate, calcium iodate, sodium selenite).

So, what have we here? For starters, in the first five ingredients, three of them are wheat—not a good start (recall the discussion on in-gredient splitting). We've previously identified meat and bone meal as being undesirable. We find salt high on the list; is that much required for health or for palatability? I'd also like to know what *natural flavor* is—specifics, please. Overall, it's not too impressive if you're looking for a healthy treat for Spot. The manufacturer uses descriptions such as "wholesome goodness" to promote this product: they haven't con-vinced me this product is wholesome or good. Here's a biscuit I would feed to Taffy: barley, beef liver, garlic, mixed tocopherols.

While I'd prefer the meat to be the first ingredient, barley is prefer-able to corn or wheat. The meat protein is identified, and garlic's role here is likely as a flavor enhancer. The ingredient list is simple, and the ingredients are suitable for a dog as an occasional snack. The problem for paropets is that simple dog snacks like this are difficult to find. Most are heavy on items such as grain or potato and contain ingredients designed to impress paropets rather than to satisfy our dogs.

In the world of dog biscuits, there are specialty products. Some prod-ucts are offered for allergic and overweight pets, so if either of those are issues in your home, discuss your needs with your pet food sup-plier. There are treats for pets with osteoarthritis that include a glucosamine/chondroitin supplement. For a serious arthritic problem I would still recommend supplementing glucosamine in addition to the treats. I used to sell shark cartilage biscuits for arthritic dogs but have discontinued those. Shark cartilage is a source of glucosamine, but there are better sources today. Besides, there's concern that some sharks have found themselves on the endangered species list due to overharvesting. Shark cartilage may be good for arthritic pets, but it's even better when left in a healthy shark.

Freeze-dried treats are among my favorites, and most are suitable for both cats and dogs. These can be made from various ingredients such as freeze-dried liver, chicken, turkey, and even fruit. Most of these products are from a single ingredient; that is, the liver package will contain only liver pieces. The freeze drying is the preservative, so other preservatives are usually absent. The meat ones are great for homes with both a cat and dog, as one treat will put a smile on every furry face. Also popular, and in a similar category as the freeze-dried products, are dehydrated treats and jerky treats. Dehydrated fish flakes and other meats, diced in small portions, are attractive to cats. Most dogs enjoy any dehydrated meat as it gives them a good chew; dehydrated sweet potatoes have proven to be winners with the canine crowd, but please keep in mind that sweet potatoes are high in calories. As some of these products are sourced from offshore (for example, China), I would exercise caution when shopping to ensure your pet is receiving a quality, healthy treat. When possible, select products made in North America; you want the package to read "Product of USA" (or Canada), not "Packaged in Canada" (or USA). Don't assume if it's a well-known North American company that the product is made here. If the country of origin for the product is not clearly identified on the package, don't buy it.

Training treats are popular; because so many are fed during a training session, providing a reward containing quality ingredients is important. Due to the quantity being fed during school sessions, training treats should be small. Even for older, trained animals, small treats are appropriate. You really don't need a big biscuit for your big dog. Generally speaking, cats and dogs care greatly that they get a treat and are less concerned with the size of the offering.

Tip: When in a training session it is important to have ready access to the rewards. If you're not happy with keeping treats loose

in a pocket, consider placing them in a small, plastic sandwich bag and then placing the bag in your pocket. The treats will be handy and your pocket will be protected from crumbs, oils, and odors.

THE TREAT TRAP

> Humans think they are smarter than their pets. Pets, I suspect, think they are smarter than humans. There's ample evidence supporting both positions.
>
> —Dave Wellock

I have two areas of concern regarding the feeding of treats to Whiskers and Spot. The first concern is overfeeding. There seems to be a logic gap here, as I have noticed many of my customers don't associate treats with food. I suppose it comes from our own attitude of not considering that quick snack as being food. We consider it a little treat or a snack, anything but food. Not only is it food, it may be extremely high in calories; read the label. If you find yourself in this group, it's time for a rethink. Your pet's treats are food. (And by the way, so are those little snacks you enjoy.)

When a customer comes into the store to discuss a weight issue regarding their pet, a portion of the conversation will involve me attempting to ascertain how many treats the pet receives on a daily basis. You'd be surprised how many paropets don't really have a good grasp on the quantity of treats doled out during the course of a day. Worse, in a multiperson household, they usually have no idea how many treats are being handed out to Whiskers or Spot by the other two-footers. Three or four medium-sized dog biscuits, to a small or medium-sized dog, can be the equivalent of a meal, or at the very least, a significant portion of a meal. To my point of view, treats are occasional pleasures, a reward for good behavior or even sometimes just as a thank you for being you.

If you're one of the guilty people freely dispensing rewards throughout the day, I suggest you stop the practice and implement some discipline—for your pet and for yourself. Spend a few minutes to determine how many treats your pet receives each day. Count them out into a measuring cup to get an idea of the volume of food those treats represent. Don't be shocked if you find it results in more food than you anticipated. Now you have two options: either reduce the number of treats you're feeding or reduce the amount of food provided in the pet's regular meal. If, for example, your dog should receive two cups of food daily, then consider it as two cups of combined food and treats. Anything else qualifies as overfeeding and will contribute to unwanted weight gain, along with all of the problems associated with obesity.

My second concern regarding treats involves planned expectations. Even more surprising than not realizing how many treats are being served, many people have no idea that their cat or dog has, in fact, trained them to deliver treats. That's right, we two-foots are the ones who are often the trainees; the pet is calling the shots. Every dog I've ever shared a roof with has known which cupboard door hides the treats. I have been led into the kitchen countless times, only to have them stare fixedly at one cupboard . . . the treat cupboard. Their quick glance in my direction holds a simple message, "Hello, stupid! What part of my body language do you fail to understand?" My cat customers advise they are also on the receiving end of this impudent message. Customers have reported to me that their pet will ask to be let outside to do its business, only to return in seconds, looking for a treat. A few minutes later, the process is repeated until the two-footer finally figures out they're being played by an unsubtle, scheming expert. There are other variations of the con that I've heard over the years, every one pointing out that we're often manipulated into doling out treats. It's probably more common than we care to admit. Are we as smart as we think, or are our pets smarter than we believe?

Both dogs and cats are creatures of habit; they have their routines and stick to them like they're federal laws. This leads us gullible two-footers into another predicament I call the Treat Trap. And we have nobody to blame but ourselves. Let's say you give Whiskers or Spot a treat just before you retire every night after watching the ten o'clock news. You've created a bad routine. On the night you decide to go to bed early, your pet will get you up for its treat at about the time when the newscast would normally finish, even if you provided a treat earlier—that's the established routine. Or this could happen. Instead of going to bed at your usual time, you stay up to watch TV. Your pet will continually pester you until you finally provide a treat. That's the routine.

Fixed treat delivery can be a bad thing. For creatures of habit, it can become an important part of their routine, one where expectations are well established and not to be violated. Other examples of the Treat Trap would include providing a treat every time the pet comes in from outside, or returns home from a walk, or does its business properly, or barks when someone knocks on the door. If you're in a Treat Trap, you'll have to slowly work your way out of it by altering the pattern. Be patient! Small steps work better than sudden, major changes to the routine. Your ultimate goal is to establish a protocol in which you provide treats, but only when you're good and ready . . . and not a second sooner. In that way, you will have regained control, escaped from the Treat Trap, and made the provision of a treat a pleasant surprise rather than an entitlement due on demand.

Question: Do cats and dogs actually need the treats we provide them, or do we have a misguided need to buy their affection?

CHAPTER 6

Pet Food's Future via My Crystal Ball

I am fond of pigs. Dogs look up to us. Cats look down on us. Pigs treat us as equals.

—Winston Churchill

What does the future hold for pet food? Good things, I'm hoping. I'm optimistic that our dogs and cats will continue to receive diets that will improve with time and advances in food technology. I'm pessimistic in that I suspect cheap, by-product-laden, grain-rich diets will, unfortunately, still be with us, dominating the market for decades to come.

The introduction of improved diets for our cats and dogs followed directly on the heels of our interest in improving our own diets. As more people commenced looking for improvements in their own foods, they also came to realize they would have healthier pets if the pets were also eating healthier foods. For people, a desire for whole foods, reduced chemicals in food, reduced processing, fewer refined ingredients, and organic products and produce has changed the dietary scenery for us, and for Whiskers and Spot. Food quality has never been more important; I sometimes tell customers, "Feed your pet or feed your vet."

It all comes down to preserving foods so they survive the journey from the farm or processor to your table (or bowl). Well, not just preserving them, but preserving them so that they end up on our table in a fresh—and safe—condition. Oxidation, as we've previously pointed out, is one enemy. Another is bacteria. E. coli, salmonella, and listeria are now common household words. Who hasn't heard media reports of widespread sickness resulting from tainted meats, fruits, and vegetables? Just this week (at the time of writing) there was a news report of hepatitis found in packages of frozen mixed berries.

We must also concern ourselves with contaminants found in pet foods. A recent contaminant, and one of the most notorious, is melamine, a chemical associated with the plastic industry. Melamine was never intended for use in foods, but it found its way into many pet foods by being incorporated into ingredients sourced from Asia. Insecticides, pesticides, and other chemicals have all made their way into pet foods.

Foods have been irradiated with X-rays, electrons, and gamma rays to kill bacteria. While it works, people have demonstrated that they don't like the concept of having their foods irradiated; they won't jump on board to have a similar treatment applied to their pets' foods. Labeling laws identifying these processes need to be updated. Detecting and preventing contaminants is more difficult to assess—virtually impossible for the consumer—and it requires great diligence on the part of those producing the foods to prevent undesirable consequences.

Commercially prepared raw diets have paved the way for a greater assortment of frozen pet foods. Pet foods that have been lightly cooked (cooked just enough to destroy bacteria, such as the baked foods discussed earlier) are becoming increasingly popular. These diets are fresher, more nutritious, and less processed than traditional kibble foods, and they are much safer than raw foods. There is little or no requirement for the addition of antioxidant preservatives, as the freezing is the preservative. Just thaw and serve. These frozen, minimally processed diets are probably the pet food of choice for concerned paropets for the near future. Still, I anticipate there is more to come where food freshness and nutrition are concerned.

One of the more promising options being investigated by food researchers is that of pressure cooking. That's misleading, so let me explain further. For this application, it's solely about pressure, with no actual cooking. Pressure cooking, as we know it in our own homes, involves placing food in a pressure cooker, turning up the heat, and cooking until the food in the pressure cooker is ready. This form of cooking may have led to the expression "don't blow your top!" as early models of these cookers were notorious for blowing their lids off when internal pressure became too intense. My mother had one of those early pressure cookers; I firmly believe I'm alive today because I avoided the kitchen whenever it was in use.

No, pressure cooking, or more appropriately "pressure preserving," as is being presently investigated, involves the application of pure pressure to foods. No heat required. The process involves placing the food in a suitable container and cranking up the atmosphere to reach one hundred thousand pounds of pressure per square inch. In comparison, an elephant sitting on your head might not feel so bad. It doesn't work for all foods such as soft fruits and leafy greens, but for those in which it does, meat, for example, you get food that is fresh, and, importantly, free of bacteria. Well, free in that there is still bacteria present . . . but they are very dead. It seems the application of intense pressure messes with bacteria's DNA and proteins, resulting in the destruction of these once-toxic organisms, thus eliminating any opportunity for them to contaminate food or compromise human or pet immune systems. After this treatment, you, along with your cat and dog, can safely eat your hamburger raw . . . if that's what you wish. I'll still opt for cooking mine . . . medium, please. Some pressure equipment is already in limited commercial food use and will likely increase in popularity as equipment costs decline and more producers incorporate it into their production systems.

I suspect this and other types of processing will eventually benefit our pet foods, allowing manufacturers to develop improved, fresher, less-processed products with a reduced need for preservatives while at the same time preventing irreparable damage to our pocketbooks. Other processes, such as laser ovens, are also being investigated.

I predict that healthy diets for cats and dogs—and people—will continue to become even more healthful in the years ahead.

On the negative side of the crystal bowl, I'm concerned about a recent trend in the manufacturing side of the pet food industry. As little as five or six years ago, one pet food giant proclaimed that healthy diets for cats and dogs would never amount to more than a niche market. The cynicism was premature. The niche, in almost no time at all, has grown from a tiny snowball to an intimidating avalanche, cutting dramatically into market share for the large, international players.

Some of the big boys have responded by introducing their own versions of healthy pet diets. Or tried! For various reasons, their intrusions into the world of healthy pet foods have pretty much proven to be a flop. I suppose it's difficult to properly feed our pets and their shareholders from the same bag or can. Then there's the issue of creditability; people who want the best nutrition for their pets have become suspicious, with good cause, of the industry giants. Still, the giants increasingly desire a slice of this growing pie: they need to protect their future.

To achieve their ends, and having failed for the most part to do so under their own flag, the industry giants are now looking to purchase the larger, established manufacturers of healthy pet diets. In the past, these corporate acquisitions have frequently led to formula alterations in the healthy food. Sometimes the ingredients are changed quickly; other times the changes are insidiously implemented over a period of time. These changes have usually proven more beneficial to the companies than to Whiskers or Spot, as the quality of the ingredients usually declines. Unfortunately, the new owners of these recently-acquired-formerly-respected brands rarely inform retailers or paropets of formula changes. The changes only come to light after the fact when customers start complaining about their pet becoming sick or rejecting a once acceptable product.

This "credibility by acquisition" is an unpleasant trend, one likely to continue as the industry giants struggle to protect their market share and shareholders. Offsetting this, smaller, innovative companies providing quality diets will continue to thrive on the strength of wholesome ingredients, improved nutrition, and an ever-growing population of informed, concerned paropets, an important group that now includes you. What the industry giants have yet to understand is that the game has changed. The ball is increasingly in the paropet's court, not theirs. Knowledge will help you retain control of the ball.

CHAPTER 7

Weighty Issues

The best thing about animals is that they don't talk much.

—Thornton Wilder

Obesity is the greatest human health problem in much of the world today. Even nations such as China and India, once unknown for obesity problems, now are experiencing the unpleasant pressure of their citizens' expanding girths. And the problem is growing worse, calorie by calorie and meal by meal.

Guess what's the largest health problem in our pet population? That's right, obesity. I suppose it's too much to expect that people who feed themselves in an irresponsible manner would do better by their pets. It's certainly not working out that way. And we can't blame the increase in the number of overweight pets on the increase in the number of overweight people. Everyone, regardless of body mass index, can be guilty here. I've been informed by countless customers that they love their pet and can't refuse them where food is concerned. My attitude is in sharp contrast to theirs. I fail to see one ounce of love in an overweight cat or dog. All I see is a lack of responsibility on the part of that paropet. There are other problems associated with excess weight, as highlighted in the following information provided in the 2011 report of the Association for Pet Obesity Prevention (APOP) (petobesityprevention.com):

The "fat pet gap" continues to widen according to the latest nationwide survey conducted by the Association for Pet Obesity Prevention (APOP).

The fifth annual veterinary survey found 53 percent of adult dogs and 55 percent of cats to be classified as overweight or obese by their veterinarian. That equals 88.4 million pets that are too heavy according to veterinarians.

"The most distressing finding in this year's study was the fact that more pet owners are unaware their pet is overweight," comments APOP founder Dr. Ernie Ward. "22 percent of dog owners and 15 percent of cat owners characterized their pet as normal weight when it was actually overweight or obese. This is what I refer to as the 'fat pet gap' or the normalization of obesity by pet parents. In simplest terms, we've made fat pets the new normal."

Perhaps even worse was the finding that the number of obese pets, those at least 30 percent above normal weight or a body condition score (BCS) of 5, continues to grow despite 93.4 percent of surveyed pet owners identifying pet obesity as a problem. The study found 24.9 percent of all cats were classified as obese and 21.4 percent of all dogs were obese in 2011. That's up from 2010 when 21.6 percent of cats and 20.6 percent of dogs were found to be obese. "What this tells us is that more and more of our pets are entering into the highest danger zone for weight-related disorders," says Ward.

Some of the common weight-related conditions in dogs and cats include osteoarthritis, type 2 diabetes, high blood pressure, breathing problems, kidney disease, and shortened life expectancy. Orthopedic surgeon, APOP board member, and Director of Clinical Research at the University of Georgia College of Veterinary Medicine, Dr. Steve Budsberg, states that the prevention of obesity needs to be at the forefront of all discussions people have about the health of their pet with their veterinarian. The body of evidence that shows the negative impact of obesity on all the body's systems is overwhelming. As an orthopedic surgeon I see, on a daily basis, the effects of obesity on dogs and cats with osteoarthritis. It is very frustrating to see how much pain and discomfort excess weight has on my patients. Veterinarians and owners have the ability to stop obesity in our pets. No animal goes to the refrigerator or the pantry and helps themselves. We enable our pets to get fat!

That's sobering! I couldn't agree more that the problem is of major proportion . . . and growing. The Pet Obesity Prevention website is worth a visit. They provide a pet weight translator, calorie chart for popular cat and dog foods, and a great deal of additional relevant information relating to this serious health problem.

Usually, it's a simple exercise to determine the cause for excess weight . . . but not always. I have a customer who, a few years ago, complained that her dog was putting on too many pounds. We went through all of the points on my checklist: overfeeding, table scraps, frequent treats, neighborly feeding, hypoactive thyroid, access to the food of other pets in the house, and more. We eliminated all plausible causes. Still, the dog continued to gain weight. She reduced his kibble to an austere survival level and monitored any and all opportunities for the dog's ability to acquire additional morsels of food. She even became a bit annoyed with me, as I was forced to continually state that the dog had to be receiving extra food from some source. After all, we don't gain weight just by breathing (although my wife claims she can gain a pound just looking at a picture of a chocolate cake). Absolutely not, was her position; the dog was not receiving extra food. It became an unpleasant situation for both of us as the dog continued to gain weight on a diet of almost starvation proportion. I was becoming nervous; if dogs could gain weight on almost no food, I'd soon be out of business.

To her credit she came into the store a few weeks later and advised I'd been right all along. The dog was receiving extra food. She arose early one morning, and when she walked into her kitchen, there was her elderly mother-in-law slyly serving the dog a large bowl overflowing with a sugary breakfast cereal. It seems the pet was happily, and secretly, on the receiving end of a large bowl of flakes every time he felt in the need of a snack, which was happening more than once each day. Worse, the more the paropet cut back the dog's food ration, the more he mooched from Grandma. Once the supply of flakes was cut off, the dog's weight began returning to normal. She was happy. I was happy. The dog was probably annoyed as hell.

The best way to avoid having your pet gain excessive weight is to monitor his or her weight on a regular basis. Prevention is the magic word here, and prevention is easier than rectifying a problem after it has developed. The simplest method for doing this is to gently press your fingertips along the ribs of the dog or cat. If you can feel ribs beneath the thin layer of the muscle and fat padding them, great! If you have to dig to find the ribs, your pet is overweight. On the other hand, if you can play a piano tune on the ribs, your pet needs more food (unless it's one of the anorexic breeds such as greyhounds or whippets). This method works well with pets whether long-haired or short-haired, cat or dog. The "fingertips on ribs" is the method I've been using for years. It works. I've never had a pet checkup during which my dog's vet has voiced any concern regarding my pet's weight, either over or under. And it only takes a couple of seconds to perform.

You can also peer down from above to see if there's an indentation at the end of the ribcage, running toward the hips. If the indentation isn't clearly defined, you need to consider reducing the chow. This method is less efficient than the fingertip system if you're dealing with a long-haired or fluffy coated pet, as the excessive fur can render a visual inspection ineffective.

By constantly monitoring your pet's physical condition for weight issues, you can marginally increase or decrease the amount of food you provide, thus solving any weight concerns before an obesity problem has an opportunity to materialize. In this case, an ounce of prevention is definitely superior to a pound of cure, especially if the pound consists of excess fat. There's an additional benefit associated with regular weight checkups. If your pet becomes too heavy or thin, and you've adjusted its food accordingly, and the condition doesn't improve or even worsens, it's time for a visit to your vet to see if there's another health issue causing the weight gain.

Tip: If your cat or dog is a bit overweight, in addition to reducing the amount of food you're feeding, consider providing a bit more of the daily chow with the morning meal, and a bit less with the evening meal. The rationale is simple. Most pets will be more active during the day, particularly if you're home all day. More walks, more following you around the house, and more visits to the backyard. Later, they'll likely fall into your unwinding routine as the evening progresses, thus requiring less food energy to make it through the night. It won't solve your problem, but it will contribute to the solution. Every little thing helps when it comes to dropping weight.

So if the worst has happened and you are now facing an overweight pet that needs to drop some weight in order to get back into shape, what do you do? The issue for your pet is the same as it is for a human. If you aren't dealing with a medical problem such as a hypoactive thyroid, then it's a case of too many calories going in and not enough out. The solution is also similar; more exercise and less food. Simple, but not as easy as it sounds, right! If it was all that easy, obesity wouldn't be a problem. If your pet is quite obese, the first step is a visit to your vet for a physical checkup, important before you implement changes that will impact its health even further. This should include a review of the pet's lifestyle, diet, and your feeding procedure, making any changes such as eliminating free-feeding or overfeeding (see Feeding Rules and Regulations in chapter 4).

Note: If you've been reducing food and providing exercise and your pet still isn't losing weight, your vet should be informed of this during the checkup. A simple blood test will determine if your four-foot has an underactive (hypoactive) thyroid. It's not uncommon, especially with mature pets. The treatment is ongoing, with vet monitoring from time to time, and the medication won't break the bank financially.

The next step is to increase your pet's exercise. This is often easier for a dog than a cat, as most dogs love their walks and are always prepared to head out on an expedition, even if just around the block. You and Spot will both benefit from a longer walk, or perhaps expanding from one walk daily to two. Keep in mind that walking to burn off excess calories is a brisk walk, not a casual stroll where you stop every few feet for an entertaining sniff at this tree or that bush. Dog parks are also great in that your dog can expend a lot of energy simply playing and running with their peers. Doggie daycares also provide opportunities for exercise through interactive play.

In addition to the above activities, there are a great many dog sports available for your pet to participate in once his or her weight reaches an acceptable level. Of course, your participation will also be required to a greater or lesser degree, depending on the sport. Here are some dog sports:

Agility
Bikejoring
Cani cross
Caniteering

Carting
Catchball/flyball
Conformation showing
Disc dog
Dog scootering
Dog hiking, pack hiking
Earthdog trials
French Ring sport
Greyhound/whippet racing
Hare coursing
Herding or stock dog hunting
Hound trailing
Junior showmanship
Lure coursing
Mushing
Musical canine freestyle; canine dressage; heelwork to music
Nose work
Obedience training
Protection sports: Schutzhund, Service Dogs of America, and Rally
    obedience
Retrieving trials
Sheepdog trials
Sighthound disc sport
Skijoring
Sled dog racing
Surfing
Terrier racing
Tracking trials
Treibball
Water work/water rescue
Weight pulling
Weiner (dachshund) racing

I confess even I don't know what's involved in some of those activities. I'll let you do the online research for those you're interested in. (I'm thinking some dogs might be geographically challenged when it comes to dog surfing.)

The point here is that there is something for nearly every dog that will provide exercise, burn off some calories, and be good fun at the same time. Think about it! Even better, the benefits will likely extend to other family members.

Those of you who have a treadmill in the home should note that a dog can be trained to use it for exercise. Basically, start with having Spot stand on the treadmill without it being turned on. Repeat this act several times, having Spot step up and off the machine. Next, position yourself to face the dog on the belt, holding its leash, and turn the treadmill on, set at its lowest speed. Let your dog stay on the belt for only a minute, and keep a supply of treats handy to be used as rewards. It may be helpful to have an assistant with you to help keep Spot in place. Don't push it. Start out with only a minute or two, gradually increasing the duration and speed over a period of days. Eventually, you should be able to have Spot use the treadmill without holding him in place with the leash. If you don't want your dog using your treadmill, there are machines designed specifically for dogs; you can find them on the Internet. Treadmills are great exercise devices for those pets in both very hot and cold climates, when temperature extremes are too severe for extended outdoor walking.

Warning: Your dog should never be tied to the treadmill or left on it unsupervised.

As most of you won't do any of the above (call me a cynic), I suggest Plan B. A ball or Frisbee in the yard or nearby park will be a good step toward shedding some excess poundage from your dog. The only challenge for you involves training Spot to return the ball or Frisbee to you on demand. If you fail in this training you'll trigger your dog's other favorite game . . . catch me if you can. This game is guaranteed to burn off excess calories . . . from each of you.

Warning: With any increase in strenuous exercise, including extending walks, you need to build up the pet's fitness level as you would for yourself. Too much, too soon can be a bad thing and result in injury or other health problems rather than healthy benefits.

Regrettably, there isn't much in the way of organized cat sports out there. All is not lost. Cat owners, too, can implement an exercise routine for their overweight pet. Heck, it's good even for a kitty that's not dealing with a weight issue. Take your cat to a pet store to fit it with a cat harness, or ask the store for instructions on measuring your cat for a harness. Usually, you only need to run a tape around the cat's chest, just behind the front legs, and take a measurement. Buy a harness that's slightly larger. Be optimistic; get an adjustable harness so that it's still useful when the cat drops that unwanted weight. The store should also be able to sell you a light leash; one about six feet long is ideal. A small retractable lead will also work.

Tip: Buy a cat harness specifically, not a small dog harness. Most cats can quickly escape from a dog harness.

Warning: Never attach a leash or tie-out to a cat's collar. Most cat collars are "breakaway" collars, designed to allow the cat to escape the collar should it become snagged on something. This safety feature of the collar will allow a cat on a leash or tie-out to escape. Also, cats do not have strong necks like dogs, so attaching something to their collar may result in physical harm to the cat.

Cats frequently object to having a harness put on them if it's something they aren't used to wearing. If you introduce them to a harness when they're a kitten, it will not be a problem later in life. Regardless, at any age adjusting to a harness is a cold-turkey process. The first time you put it on your cat, leave it on for about an hour to provide Whiskers an opportunity to adjust to the feeling. Ignore any objections and encourage them with some treats as rewards, and perhaps play some of its favorite games until it begins to feel comfortable with the harness. Continue this process once or twice daily, extending the time the harness remains on until wearing a harness is no longer an issue.

With a harness you're now able to take your cat for some exploratory walks, either around your yard or in your neighborhood. Your cat may be cautious at first, but soon it will look forward to the walks with you. You can also obtain an inexpensive cat tie-out that will allow the cat to stay outside on its own without the ability to stray any further than the end of the line. If tying Whiskers out in your yard, ensure he/she cannot access a tree or other climbable feature, or become entangled in anything such as a shrub, as this can be dangerous.

With patience, cats can often be trained to play fetch just like a dog. Chasing a small ball or other object will help maintain good physical conditioning. Also, other cat toys such as laser pointers or a feather on a string will assist in developing activity.

Tip: Here's a fun tip for exercising your cat in the house if it still retains even a bit of playfulness in its soul. Buy a small, hard, light ball. A table tennis (ping pong) ball is perfect . . . and inexpensive. Put the plug in your bathtub (no water, please). Place the cat in the tub and give the ball a toss up the rear slope of the tub. The slope will keep the ball rolling. As the cat swipes at the rolling ball, it'll keep the ball in motion. Nonstop fun! Nonstop exercise! A few minutes of that and you'll soon have a pooped pussycat.

For my customers, often the first thing they consider when dealing with an overweight pet is a weight-loss diet, or as it's sometimes called, a less-active diet. My only real objection to these diets is that I don't like to see a young kitten or puppy on a weight-loss formula. These formulas provide less nutrition than do adult or juvenile foods, and as such, I can't recommend their use for young animals except in extreme situations, and preferably on a veterinarian's instructions. Some manufacturers provide a combination diet that's labeled for weight loss and seniors. Fine! Often the issues are similar in that senior pets are frequently less active now than they were only a year or so ago, thus, while still requiring good nutrition, they need fewer calories on a daily basis.

Weight-loss diets should be used to assist in shedding unwanted pounds. Nutritionally, I don't like to see these diets used on an ongoing basis once the pet's weight has been reduced to an acceptable level. For a pet with normal weight, like Taffy, I suggest you continue feeding a regular adult diet, just less of it. Your four-foot, regardless of age, still requires good nutrition. The real problem with weight-loss diets is that they too often become a substitute for appropriate attention to weight issues and needed lifestyle changes. Your responsibility doesn't end with the provision of a weight-loss diet. You need to monitor your pet's weight frequently, control food portions, and increase physical activity.

A concerned paropet needs to pay attention to the diet's calorie content when using a weight-loss diet. Most foods do a good job of providing fewer calories per cup in a weight-loss diet versus the adult diet; some with a variance of up to a one hundred fewer calories/cup in the weight-loss version. Don't assume that holds true for all foods; the weight-loss formula of one food I checked offered only fourteen fewer calories than that provided in its regular diet. Big deal! Check the calorie information on the package, and if it's not provided, contact the manufacturer for the information. (Also see chapter 3, Calorie Content.)

Note: Rather than switching your overweight pet to a weight-loss diet, consider trying a raw, baked, or grain-free diet. These diets are lower in carbohydrates due to their higher protein content, a factor that should assist in dropping unwanted pounds.

Treats are too often a major player as a cause of pet obesity. Problems associated with misuse of treats were discussed in chapter 5, It's Hard to Beat a Good Treat. We'll briefly revisit some of that information here. Both Whiskers and Spot love their treats, and too many pet owners don't see treats as food. Many pets are skilled at manipulating their paropets into doling out treats, either through begging for tidbits when you're eating or leading you to the cupboard where the treats are stored, or both. They manipulate you by giving you The Look. The Look is that plaintive, penetrating, eye-to-eye gaze that says, more than mere words can ever convey, "If you truly love me . . ." Ignore The Look.

Treats are food. It doesn't take too many biscuits, for example, to be the equivalent of a meal. Pet treats, like human treats, are often loaded with high-calorie ingredients that contribute to weight gain. If you're dealing with an overweight pet, ask your pet food retailer for suggestions on treats that won't put on the pounds. Other great treats for preventing or reducing excessive weight are right in your home. Dogs, for example, will appreciate a raw string (snap) bean or a piece of raw carrot or other vegetable in place of a calorie-rich treat. For cats or dogs, cook a piece of chicken breast, dice it up into treat-size pieces, and feed it as a replacement for the more fattening pleasers. Keep the extra pieces in the freezer and thaw them briefly in the microwave before serving.

Again, all things in moderation! Treats are for occasional use as special rewards, not as a regular part of your pet's diet.

CHAPTER 8

Nutrition and Osteoarthritis

A cat is a puzzle for which there is no solution.

—Hazel Nicholson

Pet arthritis is a huge topic, so big I suspect books have been written on this single ailment. Arthritis is one of those discouraging diseases; discouraging because the disease has plagued the world for a long time, possibly forever. Yet in spite of our lengthy association with arthritis, it still awaits a cure. We can provide some relief for the symptoms, but we haven't yet discovered a way to eradicate the disease.

It's a disease with many victims: humans, cats, dogs, horses . . . you name it. If it's mammalian, it is probably prone to arthritis at some point. There are over one hundred different types of arthritis, and the disease, in its various forms, is the most common cause of disability in our human population, and probably our pet population as well. Osteoarthritis is the form of the disease experienced by most people and pets, and it will be the subject under discussion here.

There can be many causes for arthritis in our pets. A genetic disorder is attributed by many as the most common cause, resulting in afflicted pets inheriting the disease from a parent. A diet providing inadequate nutrition is also thought to influence the onset of arthritis, as the quality of commercial pet food was, for decades, less than desirable due to overprocessed, poor-quality ingredients. Excessive weight is certainly another contributor, as is joint injury. There is also a suspicion that generational factors working in combination may lead to the onset of the disease; specifically, generations of dogs on poor-quality diets combined with generations of poor breeding practices may be, and likely are, major contributors to the problem. It's not unreasonable to assume that osteoarthritis can result from any one—or any combination—of the above influences.

Osteoarthritis results when there is a breakdown of the cartilage, a smooth, slippery tissue protecting the ends of bones. Cartilage allows our bones to move easily without damaging each other through direct contact; in short, cartilage provides a buffer zone between moving bones. Cartilage breakdown has various causes including wear and tear due to major injuries or repeated minor injuries. Even without injuries, aging alone can be detrimental to cartilage, as wear and tear over time from normal use during aging is the reason arthritis affects seniors more than any other age group. The resulting osteoarthritis creates inflammation, pain, stiffness, and swelling in the joints of its victims. These diseased joints can become so sensitive that sufferers can actually feel discomfort from changes in barometric pressure.

Here are the signs of osteoarthritis to look for in your pet:

- Discomfort when you touch your pet's lower back or hips
- Wobbly rear end when walking
- Reluctant to walk or play
- Reluctant to negotiate stairs or jump up to a bed or chair
- Stiffness or limping, especially after resting
- Depression
- Loss of appetite
- Yelping or whimpering with some movements

Spot is more prone to arthritis than is Whiskers. I don't know why, but I do know I deal with far more dog owners for their arthritis issues than I do with cat owners. While both cats and dogs will make an effort to mask their discomfort and pain, when it comes to pretending everything is just fine, cats excel. Because cats hide their discomfort so well, the condition may progress further in our afflicted felines before their symptoms become too obvious to cover up.

There are myriad claims for arthritis cures directed at us in newspapers, magazines, and electronic media. Natural cures, medicines, gadgets, and processes abound, all claiming to eliminate our arthritic pain. Ignore them. Again, there are no cures for this disease. However, there are preventative steps that can be taken to delay the onset of arthritis and to mitigate the debilitating pain and discomfort associated with the condition.

Diet: Diet plays an important dual role here. First, good nutrition allows the body to maximize its efforts to maintain its defenses by assisting in rebuilding cartilage and combating other effects of the disease. Second, managing weight through managing the pet's diet is critically important. Overweight pets suffer far more from arthritic joints than do their thinner peers; excess weight serves to worsen arthritic conditions by putting additional stress on already stressed joints.

Exercise: Another dual benefit is found here. First, exercise assists in eliminating unwanted weight. Second, it helps keep joints limber and moving freely. For the arthritic pet, though, strenuous exercise is a bad idea. No flyball or extremely long walks, sudden stops or starts, for example. Interactive toys that encourage gentle exercise and play are great. Two short walks are now better than one long walk. For dogs, some swimming pool time often proves beneficial if done in moderation. It would also benefit a cat if you can find one who enjoys a swim.

Environmental Changes: A pet that has spent its whole life sharing your bed will still want to share your bed. Consider placing a step(s) in a location allowing access to the bed if they can no longer jump up unaided. Ramps allowing your large dog access to your SUV or truck will allow it to continue sharing rides with you. Pet beds and litter boxes might be relocated to reduce stair climbing or to avoid drafts. Ensure that comfortable bedding is provided. If your pet sleeps in a cool or damp environment, such as on a basement floor, consider relocating them to a warmer, drier location.

Physical Therapies: There are various therapies that can provide relief to arthritic pets. These include acupuncture, chiropractic, massage, laser treatment, and hydrotherapy. (The latter might not be acceptable to Whiskers.) Discuss these options with your vet.

A few years ago an elderly man came into the store to buy dog food. He looked so uncomfortable I asked if he was okay. He was fine, he claimed, just suffering from arthritis. We discussed his problem, and finally I asked him if he was taking a glucosamine supplement. He had no idea what I was talking about. I suggested he consider it, wrote it out on a slip of paper, and sent him off to a pharmacy. Three weeks later he was back. While still suffering somewhat, his arthritis no longer interfered with simple daily activities like walking as it had only weeks earlier. He was extremely grateful for my advice. He was also extremely angry with his doctor, who, in spite of his many complaints, had apparently failed to do much of anything for him beyond recommending off-the-shelf painkillers.

I did my best to make excuses for his doctor. Up until a few years ago most medical practitioners didn't know how to spell glucosamine (yes, I'm being facetious), as demonstrated by the anecdote above. In their defense, knowledge of nutraceuticals was not taught in medical school or veterinary college. Things such as herbal medicines, acupuncture, and others all fell under the heading of quackery to those practicing traditional Western medicine. Times have changed. In addition to recommending supplements such as glucosamine and chondroitin, our doctors also have an arsenal of NSAIDs (nonsteroidal anti-inflammatory drugs) available for arthritic relief.

Stores like mine have been selling health supplements such as glucosamine for many years. While lacking clinical evidence, I acquired a great deal of anecdotal support for glucosamine's beneficial impact on pets suffering from osteoarthritis. Time after time, customers would return to inform me that their pet could once again negotiate stairs, or again jump up on the bed, or now enjoyed walks, or could climb into the car's backseat, or was more playful—wonderful stories that made my day every time I heard them. Clinical studies of these supplements have proven contradictory, with some showing improvement in arthritic patients and others producing negative results. I'm satisfied it works. A dog that couldn't climb stairs on Monday but can do so on Friday doesn't require a placebo for comparative purposes.

There are three common forms of glucosamine marketed, but glucosamine sulphate is the one I recommend. Glucosamine is often sold in combination with another ingredient, chondroitin sulphate. Both are building blocks of cartilage. Glucosamine is an amino sugar, and its role in the joint is to help prevent cartilage degeneration. It won't replace damaged cartilage but may slow the process of further damage and reduce inflammation. Chondroitin sulfate provides much of the cartilage's resistance to joint compression. A loss of both glucosamine and chondroitin sulphate from cartilage has been identified as a major cause of osteoarthritis.

Many pet foods designed for seniors now contain glucosamine and chondroitin as a part of their formula. While often included in senior foods, it's sometimes in puppy formulas, especially large breed puppy foods. While I approve of its inclusion in the former, I suspect the addition of these ingredients in puppy foods is more about marketing than puppies. For puppies, it's rather like you feeding the supplement to your ten-year-old child under the premise that they may develop arthritis later in life. Who's doing that? As long as your puppy is receiving a nutritious diet, such marketing ploys are unnecessary. In any event, it won't harm the puppies and may do some good. Generally, for seniors who've developed osteoarthritis, the amount of glucosamine and chondroitin included in the diet is usually insufficient for meaningful improvement. Its bioavailability might also be compromised as a result of the cooking process used for the food. If you're dealing with an arthritic pet, reinforce the dosage with a supplement to achieve the daily levels recommended below.

Both glucosamine and chondroitin are often sold in combination with other arthritis-fighting ingredients. For example, methylsulfonylmethane, a sulphur compound usually called MSM, is a common companion ingredient. There are others. While I have no objection to the other ingredients, I'm of the opinion that the basic pair, glucosamine and chondroitin, is the one-two punch that cannot be overlooked. There are no hard and fast rules as to the appropriate daily dosage, but my rule-of-thumb dosage for pets is

Small, less than thirty pounds	500 to 1,000 mg daily
Medium, thirty to fifty pounds	1,000 mg daily
Large, fifty to one hundred pounds	1,000 to 1,500 mg daily
Giant	2,000 mg daily

When sold in combination with chondroitin, the chondroitin (and any other ingredients) will almost always be present in a lesser amount. That's okay. Let the glucosamine content be your guide rather than any of the other ingredients. The glucosamine available from a pharmacy or health food store is suitable for your pet, and any purchased from my store is suitable for you. That being said, some of mine comes complete with a yummy meaty flavor that might not please you.

Minor side effects have been listed resulting from glucosamine and chondroitin supplementation. Personally, I can only recall one dog owner reporting to me that his pet had experienced some diarrhea after taking the supplement; other than that, nothing. However, in fairness I should mention that, over the years, perhaps as many as five or six customers reported that their pet failed to experience any benefit at all. Two people using the supplement have stated the same. Those claims are likely valid as all antiarthritic measures, including prescription drugs, don't work for all people . . . or pets. I should also mention that glucosamine, to be effective in our joints, needs time to do its job. It's not a quick fix like taking aspirin for a headache. While customers have advised their pets displayed visible signs of improvement within days, I always warn them not to expect results for at least thirty days. I further advise them that if no benefit is obvious after sixty days, don't waste money on purchasing additional quantities of the supplement.

Glucosamine and chondroitin may slow down the advance of osteoarthritis, but they can't prevent the disease from developing. If not already under veterinary care for arthritis, at some point you may well be obligated to seek medical support as the disease advances. Glucosamine and chondroitin can usually be given in conjunction with prescription medications provided by your vet, but for the sake of safety, discuss this with your vet before proceeding. Veterinarians, like our doctors, now have an arsenal of antiarthritis medications at their disposal. Side effects with some of these drugs can be significant, and your vet should take care to discuss these with you in advance of starting the medications.

For cats, veterinarians have:

- **Buprenorphine:** This is a semisynthetic opioid used, among other things, in the management of chronic pain.
- **Tramadol:** A synthetic opioid analgesic. Used for treatment of severe pain. In human medications it's used for fibromyalgia, rheumatoid arthritis, and other diseases.
- **Fentanyl:** A synthetic narcotic analgesic. Used in the management of chronic pain. Approximately one hundred times more potent than morphine.

- **Meloxicam:** An NSAID. Commonly used for the treatment of canine osteoarthritis but is used off-label for other animal applications. While sometimes used with cats, feline application is controversial. (*Off-label* is the term used when a drug is administered for an application not approved by the FDA.)
- **Adequan:** Frequently used for pain treatment with horses but now being used with cats and dogs in suitably reduced dosages. Injected directly into pain sites.

For dogs, veterinarians have a wide assortment of NSAIDS in their arsenal. These are available under various names and include:

- **EtoGesic:** (Generic: etodolac).
- **Rimadyl (carprofen and its generic equivalents):** Widely used in the treatment of canine arthritis, including hip dysplasia. Can be injected. Also used for postoperative pain.
- **Deramaxx (deracoxib):** Used with dogs over four pounds. Also used for postoperative pain.
- **Metacam (meloxicam):** Injectable or oral drops.
- **Zubrin (tepoxalin).** Oral pill for severe osteoarthritic pain for dogs over 6.6 pounds.
- **Previcox (firocoxib):** Reduces pain and inflammation quickly.

NSAIDs are now the most frequently used drugs for combating the pain and discomfort of osteoarthritis in canines. Generally, they provide relief far superior to that produced by previous therapies. NSAIDs do come with an assortment of side effects, some of which are dangerous. Some of these drugs are not recommended for all breeds or sizes of dogs, as noted for Deramaxx above. Your veterinarian will be able to provide you with details. Also, NSAIDs are not recommended for canines with liver, heart, and kidney conditions. In some cases, frequent veterinarian monitoring of your pet will be required, which often includes blood work to ensure the more dangerous side effects, such as liver disease, are not developing.

Warning: All NSAIDs should only be used under veterinary supervision. NSAIDs for human use should not be used for pets without veterinary approval.

When commencing an NSAID medication program, it is important to monitor your pet for potential side effects, some of which can be serious. These effects can vary depending on which medication is being provided; any concerns specific to your pet's drug should be discussed with your veterinarian prior to starting the program. Side effects of NSAIDs include:

- Decrease/increase of appetite or thirst
- Vomiting
- Diarrhea
- Black, tarry, or bloody stools
- Lethargy
- Seizures
- Aggression
- Confusion
- Jaundice (yellowing of skin, gums, or whites of eyes)
- Altered urinary pattern: frequency, color, or smell
- Red, itchy skin

For pets, any appearance of a single one of these side effects warrants an immediate visit to your veterinarian. If the dog's stools are the concern, it may be helpful to take a stool sample to the vet for testing. I would also recommend halting medication until you and your veterinarian have an opportunity to assess developments.

Warnings: One side effect your vet may not warn you about is "feel-good injuries." Dogs that suffered from arthritic pain and are now pain free in all or part due to the drugs may overextend themselves during play or other activities, further injuring already damaged joints (sometimes severely enough to warrant euthanizing them). Paropets need to use common sense when letting these pets indulge in any physical activity.

Off-the-shelf pharmacy painkillers should not be used without veterinary approval and supervision. Acetaminophen (Tylenol and its generic variants), for example, is highly toxic to cats. The use of aspirin (acetylsalicylic acid) provides a danger of overdosing.

CANINE HIP DYSPLASIA (CHD)

There is only one smartest dog in the world, and every boy has it.

—Anonymous

No conversation on canine arthritis can be complete without a discussion on hip dysplasia. Cinnamon, my now deceased Springer spaniel, loved to play catch with a tennis ball or Frisbee. She would play until your arm was ready to fall off from throwing her toy. She, on the other hand, never seemed to tire. She could wear us out so badly that, when one family member's arm turned to lead, we'd pass the ball along to another person so her game could continue. Happy dog! Pooped people!

One day she let out a small yelp upon landing after snagging a Frisbee from the air. I put it down to coincidence at that time and thought nothing further of it. Just a bad landing, the kind every pilot dreads. However, after about the third yelping incident within a week or so, my brain finally awoke to the fact that something was amiss. Other signs, signs that I'd missed until then, began attracting my attention, such as a bit of stiffness when she got up or a slight hesitation before climbing stairs. Okay, I thought, she's a senior and some arthritis is to be expected. We added a glucosamine supplement to her diet, and that eliminated her obvious signs of discomfort. We returned to her ball games but eliminated any further Frisbee fun, concerned with the damage potential of her next hard landing. Then one day, while chasing a ground ball, she pretzeled herself when the ball took a bad bounce and was suddenly, obviously, in a great deal of pain.

Off to the vet we sped. The X-ray showed serious hip dysplasia; on a scale of one to four, Cinnamon was at least a 3.5. The glucosamine I was providing, plus Rimadyl from the vet, soon brought her back to a normal semblance of herself. However, her high-flying Frisbee catching and ball-chasing days were over, much to her dismay. Now her fun was restricted to glaring at squirrels during our walks.

I would like to interrupt myself here to point out that, over the following months, we experimented with her two medications with the following results: each time we tried to eliminate one of her treatments (glucosamine or Rimadyl), she worsened. Cinnamon's most comfortable condition resulted with the glucosamine and Rimadyl working together. While other results might be obtained with other dogs, it's worth considering a dual approach when dealing with an arthritic pet. You should discuss this dual approach with your veterinarian, and I'm unaware of glucosamine conflicting with veterinarian arthritic medications.

Hip dysplasia is found in cats, humans, and other animals occasionally. Our dogs aren't as lucky; it appears in our canine populations frequently. It's so common that the disease is one of those most frequently studied by veterinary medical researchers, as it is the usual cause of arthritis in the hip joint, a widespread health disaster for otherwise healthy dogs. Because it's so uncommon in cats, we'll leave Whiskers out of much of this conversation.

CHD is an abnormal formation of the hip socket. It's not quite that simple, though. Consider that the pelvis (hip) and femur (thighbone) operate as a ball and socket joint, with the pelvis providing the socket (acetabulum). While most dogs are born with normal hips, a genetic predisposition in some quickly leads to the abnormal development of soft tissues surrounding the joint, resulting in the ball and socket not coming together properly, a condition called subluxation. In turn, the subluxation can rapidly create a malformation of the size and shape of the ball and socket surfaces. The surrounding muscle and other tissues cannot, over time, provide proper support to an improperly embedded thighbone. Other spin-off problems can result, all leading to hip dysplasia, and eventually the development of arthritis.

Some breeds suffer more from CHD than do others. The larger breeds, such as Newfoundlands, German shepherds, and Labrador and Golden retrievers are all prone to acquiring the disease. However, while less common in small and medium breeds, it's not unusual, Cinnamon being a good example here. Purebreds are also more prone than are mixed breeds, but again, who contributed to the mixture can be a decisive factor. For some unknown reason sighthounds such as whippets and greyhounds have a low incidence of the disease. By eighteen months, hip dysplasia in most dogs with the disease will be visible with X-rays, or by newer methods such as that developed the University of Pennsylvania called the PennHIP test (research.vet.upenn.edu). Here's the introduction from their website:

PennHIP is a not-for-profit program wholly owned and operated by the University of Pennsylvania. Our mission is to develop and apply evidence-based technology to direct appropriate breeding strategies aimed at reducing in frequency and severity the osteoarthritis of canine hip dysplasia. (research.vet.upenn.edu)

PennHIP incorporates a new method for evaluating the integrity of the canine hip. It is accurate in puppies as young as sixteen weeks of age. It has great potential to lower the frequency of CHD when used as a selection criterion.

As I've inferred, some breeds are more prone to the disease than others. Here's a list of dog breeds most susceptible to the disease:

- American bulldog
- American Staffordshire terrier
- Beagle
- Bernese mountain dog
- Bloodhound
- Bouvier des Flandres
- Boykin spaniel
- Briard
- Brittany spaniel
- Bulldog
- Bullmastiff
- Chow Chow
- Chesapeake Bay retriever
- Clumber spaniel
- Coonhound
- Coton de Tulèar
- Curly coated retriever
- English setter
- English springer spaniel
- German shepherd
- Giant schnauzer
- Golden retriever
- Gordon setter
- Irish water spaniel
- Kuvasz
- Neapolitan mastiff
- Newfoundland
- Norwegian elkhound
- Old English sheepdog
- Otterhund
- Polish lowland sheepdog
- Portuguese water dog
- Pudel pointer
- Pug
- Rottweiler
- Shih tzu

- Spanish water dog
- St. Bernard
- Staffordshire terrier
- Sussex spaniel
- Welsh corgi
- Welsh springer spaniel

CHD is considered by most researchers to have a hereditary origin. This genetic picture can be complicated. If either parent has hip dysplasia, the risk of any of their offspring developing the disease is very high. The risk remains significant if even one grandparent had the disease, as the genetic carriers remain in play. By continuing to breed animals with hip dysplasia, we continue to pass along the genetic material that increases the incidence of the disease in future offspring. Conversely, responsible breeding practices will eventually impact the disease by reducing the rate of incidence. Even this can be complicated though. Even if both dogs in a breeding pair are dysplastic, their offspring may or may not show symptoms of dysplasia, and if they do, it may be in a degree greater or lesser than their parents, with the possibility of no obvious symptoms appearing at all. However, as mentioned earlier they will still be carriers of the disease, as their gene pool has become contaminated; hip dysplasia will undoubtedly appear in later generations.

As with arthritis in general, the conversation doesn't end with genetics. The spotlight has illuminated a few other potential causes for dogs with a genetic disposition toward CHD. Physical influences, for example, are often targets for investigation. These influences include excessive weight, which puts extra pressure on all joints, including the hips. Hip joint or ligament injury, especially if the injury occurs at a young age, can be a cause of arthritis. Strenuous pressure on the hip joint from excessive exercise with puppies and young dogs (such as frequent jogging) is also considered a contributor.

Exercise, however, is important for maintaining strong gluteal muscles as good muscle mass may decrease incidence of the disease. For dogs prone to the disease, regular, moderate exercise is considered more beneficial than activities that will stress joints, such as catching a Frisbee, which requires leaping, hard landings, and making rapid starts, stops, and turns. Of interest to note here is that, opposite of intense physical activity, prolonged inactivity is also on the table as a cause of the disease, as too little activity will fail to strengthen gluteal muscles.

Diet, for both quantity and quality, is considered to be another significant influence on dogs prone to CHD, especially in puppies. Owners of large breeds are particularly concerned here as rapid growth in the period up to ten months, triggered by too much food or foods with poor ingredient bioavailability, has been found to be detrimental to bone development. For this reason, many owners of large-breed puppies will feed an adult diet rather than a puppy formula as the latter usually contains additional levels of protein and carbohydrates: the adult diet should be one of good quality. Too much food is another reason I don't recommend customers free-feed their young dogs and cats after the first few weeks. A report appeared recently noting that in one study, Labrador retriever puppies fed free-choice for three years had a much higher incidence of CHD than their littermates who were fed the same diet but in an amount that was 25 percent less than that fed to the free-choice group.

Clearly, the results from the Labrador puppy feeding trial are significant, demonstrating that dogs may develop hip dysplasia generated by nothing more complicated than a misguided feeding program. Obviously, they will be healthier on a controlled, nutritious diet. I suspect most of our cats and dogs—and their two-footers—will have longer, healthier lives if they're one pound underweight versus one pound overweight.

FATTY ACIDS AND ARTHRITIS

> Animals are such agreeable friends—they ask no questions, they pass no criticisms.
>
> —George Eliot

Omega-3 fatty acids, those beneficial fat compounds commonly found in some plant oils such as flax seed and fish oils such as salmon, have been clinically determined to benefit sufferers of rheumatoid arthritis, a form of arthritis not prevalent in our pets. Some recent studies now show that there are significant benefits to be gained by using it for people and pets suffering from osteoarthritis, both for preventing the onset of the disease and for mitigating its effect on our joints. Another plus is that it should be safe to use in conjunction with any other arthritis treatment being provided, such as glucosamine or NSAIDs, but if you're concerned, discuss it with your veterinarian before proceeding.

Omega-3 (alpha-linolenic acid) is one of the two essential fatty acids (EFAs), the other being omega-6 (linoleic acid). They are called "essential" because the body cannot manufacture them on its own and because they play a fundamental role in several physiological functions. (There are other fatty acids, but these two are identified as essential.) Most of us, and our pets, receive adequate amounts of omega-6 from dietary sources: most vegetable oils, for example, provide omega-6, as do nuts, cereals, and even fast foods. This is often not the case with omega-3, as all of us would likely benefit from eating more foods that contain the ingredient. There are both plant and fish sources for this fatty acid, as mentioned. While both sources provide omega-3 fatty acids, all omega-3s aren't identical . . . or equal. Clinically, oil sources from coldwater fish species such as salmon are considered superior to plant sources such as flax and hemp seed oils.

My recommendation for any pet suffering from arthritis is to include a good-quality omega-3 fish oil supplement in their daily diet. You can obtain a supply from most pharmacies, health food stores, and many pet supply retailers. The product usually comes in capsule or liquid form. The latter is often easier to get into a pet as it can be added directly to their food. A caution with oils is warranted here: never introduce too much oil too quickly into your pet's diet as you may generate very soft or loose stools for a day or two. Instead, start with about a quarter of the recommended dose and build up to a full dose over several days. With fussy eaters, particularly cats, it may be wise to start with only a couple of drops for a day or two, gradually building up to a full dose.

Omega-3 will appear again in the following chapter on allergies.

SURGERY CONSIDERATIONS

Cats are rather delicate creatures and they are subject to a good many different ailments, but I have never heard of one who suffered from insomnia.

—Joseph Wood Krutch

When dealing with dysplasia most veterinarians will recommend therapies that include painkillers and anti-inflammatories such as NSAIDs; as well, they may suggest dietary supplements such as glucosamine and omega-3 fatty acids. Vets may also discuss other important considerations, such as altering your pet's lifestyle by eliminating strenuous exercise or play and placing overweight pets on a controlled diet in order to shed the unwanted pounds. In some cases they may suggest the option of surgery. Because the disease is so prevalent, corrective surgery techniques are routinely performed to address the various conditions associated with it. The following summarizes the available surgery options:

Femoral Head Ostectomy (FHO): This fairly simple procedure can be used on many animals but has proven most successful with cats and small dogs that are not overweight. Usually, one hip is done and allowed to heal and become functional before the other hip is treated. When the head of the femur becomes roughened, or rough-edged, it is removed surgically. The remaining portion of the femur produces a false joint; bone-to-bone contact is eliminated through the development of fibrous scar tissue. There is usually some loss in mobility and a change in gait, with most pets managing nearly normal mobility function after healing. Pain is all but eliminated with this procedure. It is critical that pets that have undergone this surgery not gain postoperative weight and retain a desired weight for the remainder of their lives. Following surgery, early physiotherapy is required, as the scarring might otherwise restrict future mobility. Slow walks of short duration are encouraged.

Triple Pelvic Osteotomy (TPO): The name stems from a requirement to make three incisions in the pelvis. This surgery is usually restricted to younger dogs under one year old with minimal or no signs of arthritis. Candidates will be physically examined and X-rayed to determine their suitability for this surgery. Where both hips require TPO, some surgeons elect to do them in a single, long procedure; others prefer to work on one at a time, allowing weeks or even months between surgeries. This is a major surgery, and pets undergoing it must have six weeks of confined rest following the completion of the procedure. After six weeks dogs will be able to walk well.

The objective of TPO is to alter the orientation of the shallow hip socket (acetabulum) to allow a better fit with the head of the femur. This increases the stability of the joint and helps to minimize the development of arthritis as the dog gets older. The new socket will be held in place with screws and a special plate. When corrected early enough, potential arthritic damage is minimized; this should be the only surgical procedure necessary.

DARthroplasty: Some young dogs may have a socket (acetabulum) that's too shallow for a TPO but are too young to be ideal candidates for a total hip replacement (THR). This new procedure may be just the ticket. During the operation, bone is harvested from the dog's own pelvis and then used to create a shelf of bone over the rim of the socket, in essence creating a deeper socket. This bone fuses in its new position and prevents the head of the femur from sliding in and out of the shallow socket. This is a relatively new technique, but good results have been reported.

Total Hip Replacement (THR): If the above procedures are not applicable for reasons of age or a pelvic socket condition that precludes remedial work, then returning the dog to a normal function may require replacing damaged joints with artificial ball and socket joints of stainless steel or titanium. The ideal candidates here are at least two years old so that their bones are sufficiently mature for accepting the implants. An existing arthritic condition in the joint is not usually a deterrent to this surgery. Like TPO, this intrusive surgery requires that pets undergoing it must have six weeks of confined rest following completion of the procedure. After six weeks dogs will be able to walk well but should start with slow, short, controlled walks, gradually building to longer walks.

New for Tomorrow: In the future, new procedures for reducing the impact of osteoarthritis, or even better, defeating it altogether, will hopefully be discovered. One of these—showing great promise—is stem cell therapy. Should a breakthrough occur as a result of stem cell research, millions of mammals—dogs, cats, horses, and humans—will be incredibly grateful.

CHAPTER 9

Nutrition and Allergies

If I have any beliefs about immortality it is that certain dogs I know will go to heaven, and very, very few people.

—James Thurber

An allergy develops when a foreign substance (an allergen) activates the immune system. If your pet suffers from an allergy, then it's important to understand that their immune system is under attack; it has been compromised to the point in which it is overreacting to a substance, even one as common as a food ingredient. Allergies are not age related. Your pet may develop symptoms at any point in its life. The weaker the immune system, the more prone it will be to an allergen. An allergy is not an equal-opportunity problem; two littermates living in the same home and eating the same food may have different responses, with one developing a serious allergy and the other totally unaffected. Most allergies can be categorized into one of two groups, food or environmental. Environmental allergies can be caused by inhalants such as air pollution and pollens, or by contact with biting insects, household chemicals, plastics, and fabrics, or from some drugs such as penicillin or sulfonamides. Regardless of the cause, the symptoms that materialize can be the same.

The role of food in causing allergic responses can be complicated, as numerous factors may be involved. Consistent overfeeding can lead to immunity problems. Overly processed ingredients may create a reaction. Yeast and fungi contaminants, and trace amounts of pesticides, herbicides, and drugs contained within the food, might prove problematic for a hypersensitive pet. Stress can compromise the digestive system, which in turn may compromise the immune system. Genetic susceptibilities to certain ingredients may be passed from parent to offspring. And most commonly, a specific food ingredient may create an allergy problem.

With cats and dogs, allergy symptoms frequently appear as skin and coat problems. Humans have sweat glands over much of their bodies, and these glands can assist in ridding the body of toxins. Cats and dogs, on the other hand, have very few sweat glands, and, as a result, are less efficient at secreting toxins, thereby turning their skin into an allergy signboard. Common symptoms of an allergy attack include:

Dermal Responses:

- Hot spot (a patch of inflamed skin, reddish, itchy)
- Excessive paw licking
- Irritated rear end (anus, genital areas)
- Rash and itchy skin, skin sores and dry, flaky (dandruff) skin
- Biting/chewing at root of the tail and other body areas
- Excessive body odor
- Inflamed ears, chronic ear infections
- Excessive hair loss, dull and brittle coat, bald spots
- Discolored skin (grayish)
- Runny, goopy eyes

Respiratory Responses:

- Bad breath
- Wheezing, coughing, sneezing, panting

Digestive Responses:

- Diarrhea, constipation, vomiting

Systemic Responses:

- Swelling of the face or throat, and in severe cases, anaphylactic shock

Any cat or dog can become a victim of an allergy; it's the luck of the draw. However, some pets may be unluckier than others. While cats do suffer from allergies, the incidence of the problem is, from my experience, much lower in our feline population than in the canine crowd. This is borne out with manufacturers—influenced by demand—producing a much smaller selection of allergy diets for cats than dogs. Furthermore, allergies in the cat population appear to be quite random, as I'm unaware of any breed-specific tendencies toward the problem. Not so with our dogs. Among dogs, the following breeds seem to be more prone to contracting allergies, be it food or environmental, than do others.

Boxer
Chihuahua
Cocker spaniel
Dachshund
Dalmation
German shepherds
Golden retriever
Irish setter
Labrador retriever
Lhasa apso
Miniature schnauzer
Poodle
Shar pei
Shiba inu
Shih tzu
Some terriers: Westies, fox, Yorkie, Cairn, Scottish, Wheaton, and
   Boston

I hate to admit this, but pet allergies have, over the years, been very good for my business. They must also be good for the pet food industry as a whole because, increasingly, the number of allergy diets appearing on the market continues to grow. Allergy diets, or as they are now beginning to call them, "limited ingredient diets," are commonly available from pet specialty retailers like me, as well as through veterinarian clinics.

When I first took over my business, there were few diets specifically targeting allergies. If your pet had an obvious allergy to a food, there were alternatives available, but these alternative diets were usually limited to lamb and rice formulas, with a quality not much better than other products on the shelf. Still, it moved Spot or Whiskers from a corn-based chicken protein meal to a rice-based lamb protein meal, and sometimes that did the job. Times have changed. Here's an example of a limited ingredient (allergy) feline diet: peas, salmon meal, pea protein, salmon, canola oil, flaxseed, and natural flavor (author's note: to eliminate redundancy, I've excluded the vitamin/mineral supplement package included with this formula).

You will note that the only meat source is salmon and the only carbohydrate source is provided by peas, both not normally an ingredient in traditional cat foods. The salmon, canola oil, and flaxseed will all provide omega-3 fatty acids to assist the cat's body in dealing with allergies. The ingredient list is short (limited) because, when dealing with a potential food allergy, you want to eliminate as many ingredients as possible, as each additional ingredient could prove to be an allergy cause.

A few weeks after introducing the first high-quality food into the store, a woman came in seeking a food to help her troubled dog, a young German shepherd. The dog was losing hair to the point of being bald in spots, and what hair remained was brittle and dull. Worse, it had a rash over much of its body, with hot spots frequently breaking out. The condition had been ongoing for almost a year, slowly worsening from month to month, and the poor thing was obviously miserable within its own skin. Frequent visits to two veterinarians and changing diets innumerable times had failed to solve the dog's problems.

I had introduced this product into my store at the request of a customer who was driving a great distance to another community to purchase it. It was a risky proposition, as the product sold for over $20 more per bag than anything else on my shelves. As the owner of the troubled German shepherd had tried nearly every brand of dog food available in our community, with no beneficial results, she opted to buy a bag of the new food. She was back in two weeks, happily advising that the rash was clearing up and the hot spots were appearing less frequently and vanishing much faster. By the end of a month the shedding had ceased and some fuzz was appearing on the bald spots. Within two months she had a brand new dog; they never looked back.

Now I had an allergy diet. Even better, I also had a customer who was well known in the local dog community—a customer who unhesitatingly promoted my store with its wholesome food. New customers were soon finding me. It's interesting about word-of-mouth advertising; when it's working for you, it's wonderful. It is, however, a double-edged sword that can also work against you if you're not careful. Fortunately, the verbal advertising now working for me was totally positive; to this day we rely heavily on our customers to promote our business.

In those days, veterinary science was of the opinion that the majority of pet allergies were environmentally caused by sources such as household chemicals, pollen, and pollution. In that scenario, food-related allergies accounted for an insignificant third, or less, of allergy cases. My experience with allergic pets was just the opposite, as we successfully used diet changes to cure the majority of allergic dogs and cats that came to us. While I frequently wondered why the local vets weren't solving more of the problems being brought to me, I eventually concluded that the veterinary community was handicapped by the preconceived ideas taught them while in college, ideas that, from my viewpoint, were erroneous. In their defense, food, as it relates to health, was not often taught to veterinarians (or our human doctors) as a part of their education. (At one seminar on pet health and nutrition I attended, a young veterinary student in the audience told us most of the information on pet nutrition she and her peers had received was provided by guest lecturers representing major pet food companies.) The few vets that seemed to be on my side of the table were those who, following graduation, began thinking outside of the box, often eventually identifying themselves as holistic veterinarians.

I came to the issue of food-related allergies with no preconceived ideas. Truthfully, in the beginning I was so ignorant regarding the problem you could rightfully claim I lacked any ideas on the topic at all, preconceived or otherwise. Eventually, I became so successful at clearing up allergy problems that I started to worry I was becoming an embarrassment to my local veterinarian community. After all, they had had a crack at curing these pets prior to them arriving on my doorstep I wanted the vets as allies, not enemies, but it was an awkward time. To their credit, the vets accepted my successes with grace; eventually some even directed clients to my store for specific diets. There's been improvement on another front: the veterinarian colleges must be doing a better job as graduating veterinarians today seem to be facing food-related health issues with more open minds.

Tip: If you suspect your pet has developed an allergy, your first stop should be your veterinary clinic, not a pet supply store. Some allergy symptoms may be indicative of other diseases and not be allergy related at all. Having a proper medical diagnosis is an important first step. If the problem is suspected of being a food allergy, you will likely find superior products available in pet food stores. Find a store capable of providing sound advice.

Don't get me wrong here. All pet allergies cannot be solved with a change in diet. There are, in fact, many environmental triggers out there having nothing to do with food, and not all are obvious such as tree or grass pollen. Many can come from within the home, such as food storage, air, and water quality. Adding to the confusion, it appears that in some instances, a pet with an immune system compromised by one type of allergy, let's say environmental, may be more susceptible to a potential food allergy, or vice versa.

In order to avoid sounding too cocky, I'm the first to admit I've failed many pets in attempting to clean up their allergies. The victories are sweet, but it's the failures I think about most often. Dealing with a pet's allergies is not a simple matter. I always tell customers that solving the problem is, at best, a crapshoot, a guessing game. For starters, Whiskers and Spot can't talk. Well, they can't speak languages we can understand, like English, Spanish, or Mandarin. Fortunately, their human owners are prepared to fill the communication gap. I strongly believe that much of the success I've enjoyed in this area comes from conversations with paropets prior to actually selling them anything, as I'm hesitant to sell them something until I have a reasonable idea of what it is we're dealing with. I ask questions—lots of questions. "How old is your dog?" "What breed is it?" "When did the problem begin?" "Is it worse more at some times than others?" "What foods have you tried?" "Are the cat's food and water dishes made of plastic?" "Are there hot spots (or hair loss, or bad breath, or body odor)?" "How do you store the food?" And lots more! I can sometimes spend up to thirty minutes asking questions and discussing the answers. The funny thing is, regardless of how frivolous some of the questions may appear I've yet to have a customer resent the questioning; most seem to appreciate my interest in their problem. Sometimes I even apologize for asking so many questions.

There are times when few questions are required, as you can leap to a reasonable conclusion based on minimal information or evidence. I recall a couple coming into the store one time with a hair-loss concern for their German shepherd cross. As the dog was in the back of their pickup truck, I invited them to bring him inside for a closer look. I was observing when the dog jumped down from the bed of the truck. The brief physical act of jumping down triggered a cloud of hair flying from its body, the cloud clearly visible to me standing over twenty feet away. It was a jaw-dropping sight. Do you recall the Pig-Pen character in the Peanuts comic strip? Pig-Pen always appeared amid a cloud of dust and dirt. This could have been Pig-Pen's dog if flying hair was dirt. When the dog came into the store I could effortlessly pull handfuls of hair from his body; he visibly dropped hair every time he moved. The poor thing was a walking disaster. It was so bad I had to vacuum the floor after they left.

I had but one question for them as the dog entered the store: "What are you feeding him?" He was dining on one of the cheapest, lowest quality dog foods available at that time (and still available today), a food predominantly consisting of unidentifiable meat and grain by-products. And when I say cheap, I mean dirt cheap. There is no exaggeration here when I say that a bag of pigeon feed was more expensive than a bag of this particular dog food. I know, because I had one customer using pigeon feed at that time. This dog didn't require a top-of-the-line diet or an allergy diet, just a better-quality diet. These folks couldn't afford a top food anyway, as their pickup looked to be in worse shape than their dog. I sold them an appropriate bag of food and sent them on their way. They never returned, so I don't know the outcome. I could only hope they took my advice and continued feeding the dog something of better quality, as it didn't deserve to be fed so poorly. The problem here is that many people want a pet . . . even if they can't afford to feed it decent food. Sadly, they also have children and can't afford to feed them properly either.

The purpose in asking so many questions is simple: eventually, the customer often will unknowingly identify the probable solution. Even then, as I said above, it's a guessing game. The questions provide us with a starting point. Then it often becomes a process of elimination. We try one diet for four to six weeks and monitor results; if there's progress in reducing the symptoms, we will stay with the diet for an additional two or three months, monitoring constantly. If there's no progress, we move to another diet and start over again. I try to make it clear to the customers that the program is not about me selling food; it's about clearing up a health problem. Whether you're buying an allergy food from a store like mine or from a veterinarian, the food should provide a benefit within a reasonable time, about two months.

Note: I've had customers who continued buying a food for their allergic pet without advising me they aren't getting a benefit. Others have done the same with a vet diet. If the diet doesn't deliver a benefit, don't stay with it, as you're defeating the purpose. Drop it and try a different food; there are lots of options.

The problem with most allergies is, even if you solve them, there's a good chance you'll never know what specifically triggered the symptoms. If the diet is associated with the allergy, immediate suspicion usually falls to the main ingredients, such as the corn, wheat, or the meat protein. Those may or may not be the culprits. Most foods have a variety of ingredients beyond the primary ones. All you need is one single ingredient, present even in a small quantity from well down the ingredient list, and you can create an allergic response. Sometimes the response happens quickly; other times the symptoms may take days, weeks, or even months to appear as the small amount of toxin slowly accumulates within the body until symptoms become obvious.

My initial approach in working with an allergic pet is to determine if the root of the problem lies with environmental causes or is food related. An important question here relates to the frequency of symptoms. Are the symptoms present all of the time, day in and day out, or do they come and go on a seasonal basis? If the latter, then it's likely the allergy's cause may be environmental, as food allergies aren't subject to seasonal influences. With food allergies, you eat every day and you suffer every day. This is not a rock-hard truth, though, as indoor environmental causes that the pet lives with daily can and will trigger ongoing symptoms. Still, it's a fairly safe bet to go with a food allergy if the problem is consistent on a daily basis because indoor environmental causes aren't that common; certainly not as common as food allergies.

Once we've targeted food as the culprit, the next step is to determine which diet option may be best for an initial trial run. This is an important step for me as a bad selection might result in a continuation of the problem, or even a worsening of it, and perhaps a lost customer. None of those outcomes is desirable. Fortunately, most of the allergy diets I now carry usually prove beneficial. We may not get a total turnaround, but any improvement in lessening the severity of the symptoms is progress. If we've altered the symptom's impact, we know we're on the right track.

Certain food ingredients have been more associated with allergies in our pets than others. These include:

For Cats:	For Dogs:
Lamb	Beef
Beef	Lamb
Turkey	Chicken
Corn ingredients	Corn ingredients
Seafood	Wheat ingredients
Soy ingredients	Soy ingredients
Wheat ingredients	Dairy products including whey
Dairy products	

Remember, while this list provides the "big ticket" items for allergy triggers, the actual guilty party may be some other ingredient. It's not surprising to see dairy products on both lists. I believe I pointed out in another chapter that almost all cats and dogs are lactose intolerant, at least to bovine products. That cute kitten licking up a saucer of milk may be in trouble. A small amount of dairy products from time to time won't likely cause a problem. Too much dairy product at one sitting, or small amounts provided frequently over time, may prove detrimental. If you insist on providing dairy products to your pets, look for those in your supermarket that are lactose free.

Obviously, if you're dealing with a food allergy, you want to avoid diets with any of the above ingredients. That's where allergy/limited ingredient diets come into play. A typical allergy diet will include a single meat protein, ideally from a source Whiskers or Spot have not previously experienced. These will incorporate meats such as duck, fish, pheasant, venison, bison, kangaroo, or others. There will also be a single carbohydrate source, again one not normally experienced by the pet. Common in this group are potato, sweet potato, rice, green pea, and oatmeal. Typically, the remaining ingredients will be the usual cocktail of vitamin and mineral supplements necessary for sustaining good overall health.

Note: Unlike in the anecdote provided above in which the problem was fairly obvious, you should understand that sometimes it's difficult to differentiate between a pet suffering from food allergies or simply from a nutritionally deficient diet. If undecided, often I'll put them on an allergy diet until symptoms lessen or vanish, then see if we can wean them back onto a normal diet, but one of improved quality. Due to the limited ingredient profile of allergy diets, I prefer to not keep a pet on them unless there's no other recourse.

We have also experienced success in treating allergies with the new diets that have been appearing in the past few years. As mentioned, processed foods alone, regardless of ingredients, may be allergy triggers. Frozen raw or baked meals and dehydrated whole foods have helped some of our cats and dogs return to good health when allergy diets have failed. Still, I'll initially try a couple of allergy diets first. If they fail to eliminate or reduce the symptoms satisfactorily, then we'll often implement a feeding trial with one of these newer foods. As I've stated, it's always a guessing game, and you never know what will work.

There are numerous other steps we can take to clear up an allergy problem. Most deal with the pet's immediate environment. While minor, there's always the chance one of them may prove to be the allergy trigger. All of them at one time or another has caused allergies in pets that I've dealt with. Some of these are:

- **Plastic dishes:** Plastic bowls and dishes are fine for most cats and dogs. You should ensure that they are made from plastic designed for food use. Regardless, a small number of pets seem to develop allergy symptoms that can be attributed only to their plastic dinnerware. As a precaution, I usually recommend changing the food and water dishes from plastic to ceramic or stainless steel. Ensure they're washed after each use.
- **Drinking water:** Like plastic bowls, tap water is perfectly fine for most pets as it is for most people. Until we've resolved the allergy problem, I recommend using filtered or bottled water. A customer

had a twelve-year-old border collie with allergies so severe they contemplated putting the dog down. We implemented several new procedures, including an allergy diet, and cleaned up all but one of the symptoms in six weeks. The remaining problem was a loud gurgling from the bowels when the dog was lying down. Having tried everything else, we changed its water source and that remaining problem vanished in a day. The dog remained perfectly healthy until old age caught up with it.

- **Pet bedding:** Wash your allergic pet's bedding frequently. Also, note that some fabrics may cause allergies in some pets. If problems persist, it may be wise to provide other bedding for a few months to see if symptoms improve.

- **Chews:** Favorite chew treats can be responsible for allergies, especially if they contain dyes. Rawhide chews and meat chews such as bully sticks should be discontinued until allergy symptoms improve. Also remove plastic toys, as some plastics can be harmful.

- **Treats:** If you're putting your pet on an allergy diet, provide an allergy treat at the same time. Be leery of feeding popular soft, chewy treats as they may contain every undesirable food ingredient and chemical preservative you've ever heard of, along with unnecessary salt, sugars, and dyes. They bring the definition of "junk food" to a new, lower level. A piece of carrot usually makes a dog smile and will not likely impact its allergy. A few pieces of their kibble will normally be well received by Whiskers and Spot as a safe treat at this time.

- **Yard/house chemicals:** Several years ago someone noted a significant increase in a cancer, soft tissue sarcoma, in children. Someone else noted a similar relationship in cats and dogs. The finger pointed to lawn treatments with both herbicides and insecticides, one reason many communities have banned or restricted the application of these products. The problem lies with the fact that children often play barefoot in the yard. Our pets, of course, are always barefoot. Chemicals absorbed through the skin can be toxic; trace amounts can create allergic responses. I always caution pet owners to protect pets from these yard conditions. While most household chemicals and cleaners are safe for you, remember that your pet's feet aren't protected with shoes, slippers, and socks.

ALLERGIES AND OMEGA-3 FATTY ACIDS

Dogs are my favorite people.

—Richard Dean Anderson

In the prior chapter on osteoarthritis, we discussed the arthritis-related benefits derived from supplementing the pet's diet with an omega-3 fatty acid (alpha-linolenic). Not only does it have a proven track record in helping reduce arthritis symptoms, it also provides a benefit for those pets suffering from some types of allergies. I frequently recommend an omega-3 supplement if the pet suffers from:

- Skin rash or discolored skin
- Hot spots and open/slow healing sores
- Dandruff
- Dull, brittle coat
- Excessive hair loss
- Excessive body odor

As previously mentioned, we usually receive sufficient quantities of omega-6 (linoleic acid) from our diet. It's a requirement for healthy skin and hair, among other things. Looking at the list immediately above, you will note they are all skin and hair concerns. The problem is that as soon as the skin is injured in any way, that is, a scratch or hot spot, omega-6 acts as an inflammatory agent, further irritating the injury. Omega-3 fatty acid, on the other hand, brings a unique talent to the aid of injured skin by acting as an anti-inflammatory, thus countering much of the negative impact of omega-6 on the injury. By helping reduce the inflammation at the injury site, it reduces itchiness and assists in a speedier healing process.

Tip: I also recommend using an omega-3 supplement with cats, especially the long-haired breeds who often suffer from hairball problems; a reduction in shedding will reduce hairball production.

DIGESTIVE ENZYMES

If a dog jumps into your lap, it is because he is fond of you; but if a cat does the same thing, it is because your lap is warmer.

—Alfred North Whitehead

Another supplement I recommend when dealing with food-related allergies is a good digestive enzyme product. Poorly digested food can create toxins in the intestinal tract that can stress the immune system, and in turn generate allergy symptoms and other problems. Digestive enzymes assist in breaking down our food more efficiently. While younger animals seem to possess sufficient digestive enzymes in their system, middle-aged and senior pets may not be so lucky. (Have you ever noticed how gassy senior humans can be?) For older pets, these enzymes are a good idea, and they are inexpensive and easily added to the meal as they normally come in a powder form. Digestive enzymes are available from pet supply stores, health food stores, and pharmacies. Raw fruits and vegetables are also good sources of digestive enzymes, but remember, only provide these food items in small amounts.

OTHER ALLERGY PROBLEMS

> Heaven goes by favor; if it went by merit, you would stay out and your dog would go in.
>
> —Mark Twain

Up to this point we've discussed food-related allergies in detail and touched on contact allergies. Additionally, there are two other categories that require mention, flea bite allergy and allergic inhalant dermatitis.

Flea bite allergy: Many cats and dogs have little or no reaction to flea bites, while others can become seriously miserable as a result of just a few bites. It's a similar story with people; a dozen mosquito bites barely bother me, but a single mosquito bite can drive my wife crazy. The reason for this may lie in the robustness of each animal's immune system. Pets susceptible to other allergies, such as food or air pollution, may react more strongly to flea bites than do their fellows.

Allergic reactions to flea bites usually materialize rapidly. If your pet suddenly commences scratching or chewing itself, examining them for fleas would be the first step to take. The flea bite marks themselves will be quite tiny—like little pinpricks—but there may be a small circle of inflammation surrounding the bite sites. On some hairier pets, identifying flea bite marks, or even live fleas, can be difficult. On lighter-colored pets look for flea dirt (poop), which resembles a small pinch of pepper near the base of hairs, or use a flea comb to capture the evildoers. If fleas are found, then you've probably found the cause of the sudden onset of scratching and chewing. For a pet not suffering greatly from the problem, I would apply flea drops or a flea collar immediately. For a pet that's suffering a great deal, I'd want to rid it of fleas very quickly with a flea bath, followed by applying drops or a collar so that new fleas will die quickly following contact with your pet.

I would also give Spot or Whiskers an omega-3 supplement to assist in reducing itchiness and inflammation. Furthermore, for those suffering greatly, an antihistamine may be helpful. The antihistamine Benadryl is, I know, considered safe for both cats and dogs. If the pet is on other medications (or not), you may want to discuss antihistamines with your veterinarian prior to administering the drug.

Warning: Not all antihistamines are necessarily safe for pets, so if you are using any other product I strongly urge you to discuss it with your veterinarian in advance.

If using Benadryl, the usual recommended dose is 1 mg per one pound of pet, given every eight hours (three times daily). Thus, a forty-pound dog would receive a 40 mg dose once every eight hours to a maximum of 120 mg in each twenty-four-hour period.

It's worth noting here that good nutrition does play a role in dealing with insect bites. Good nutrition supports a healthy immune system. Healthy pets are less reactive to insect bites and are less attractive to fleas in the first place.

Allergic inhalant dermatitis: This allergy involves breathing in an antigen. An antigen is any substance that causes your immune system to produce antibodies against it. For inhalant antigens, this would include pollens, dust, dust mites, mold, and dander. In humans, a classic inhalant antigen results in what is commonly called hay fever. It becomes *allergic inhalant dermatitis* when the immune system is sufficiently compromised by the inhaled antigens to result in an itchy or inflamed skin, like hot spots or a rash. It is estimated that up to 30 percent of pets may be affected at different times throughout their lives. The most common areas affected are the face, feet, front legs, ears, and armpits.

The cause(s) of this allergy can be difficult to determine and requires professional investigation, usually with a procedure known as an intradermal test, informally called a scratch test. Antigens found in the pet's environment are introduced to the skin in solutions of varying strength, and then the injection sites are monitored for reactions. If the testing has identified a specific substance as the culprit, every effort should be made to eliminate or reduce it from the pet's environment. This is relatively easy to accomplish if you're dealing with a food ingredient, chemicals, or a fabric. Airborne allergens are another problem, one often more difficult to cope with. Room air filters may help with allergens such as mold and dust mites.

Subject to the severity of your pet's reaction, your veterinarian may also recommend relieving the symptoms with a corticosteroid such as prednisone, or antihistamines such as Benadryl. With this type of allergy attack, antihistamines often fail to provide significant improvement. Steroids are usually effective with most allergens but are recommended for short-term application only, as side effects can be many and serious. The adverse reactions my customers' pets have experienced from steroid use include excessive hunger/weight gain, nervousness, and changes in personality. The downside is that both steroids and antihistamines are only bandages, not cures. The relief they provide is temporary at best. Over the years I have witnessed too many pets, predominantly dogs, on what I call a "prednisone cycle." When they're on the steroid, the symptoms are diminished and the pet is relieved of the agonies caused by the allergy; when the pet is off the steroid, the problem returns, often quickly, and the cycle commences all over again, on and off like a light.

Steroid use isn't restricted to allergic inhalant dermatitis problems, however. It will often be prescribed for any allergy condition, especially if it materializes as skin problems. I don't like steroids, and I'm sure most vets aren't happy providing them, especially on a repeat basis. However, it's truly a case of being stuck between a rock and a hard place. Yes, they provide relief, but only temporarily.

Dealing with an allergic pet on steroids is a challenge for me. While on steroids, it's impossible to determine if other changes—such as switching to an allergy diet—are having any impact on the condition. In this situation, the best I can do is change the diet and let the steroid prescription run its course. Hopefully, at the end of the process, if the food is providing a benefit, we can eliminate any future need for steroids, or at least dramatically stretch out the interval between applications.

Immunotherapy is another option now being used. Once the allergen has been identified, usually through intradermal testing, a series of shots using that allergen is administered over several years with the purpose of desensitizing Whiskers or Spot. The procedure has a good success rate, but it should be noted that it doesn't work on all animals, and in some cases the health improvement may be minimal. If successful, the benefits can last for years. There is an advantage to commencing the program at an early stage with younger pets, or if older, as soon as possible after the onset of the problem.

Runny, goopy eyes: Surprisingly, most paropets don't see this as an obvious allergy problem. There is always a bit of eye weeping; that's to be expected. When the weeping becomes excessive, it's a message that all is not right, and it is a warning that a more serious problem may be developing. Although the cause for this condition, like other allergies, can be either food or environmental, I have found that food is often the culprit. If you're feeding kibble, transition your pet to a good-quality allergy diet for thirty days. If results aren't satisfactory, try a second kibble diet for another month, preferably one with a low- or no-grain content. If still unsatisfied, I would suggest a baked, or even raw, diet for an additional month. Once the problem returns to normal, you can be confident that not only have you eliminated a minor condition but also you've likely prevented a more serious allergy problem from developing.

Human nature demands answers; sometimes there are none. We often never know the cause of an allergy attack. If you can prevent it from recurring in the future, be grateful.

VACCINATIONS

If you can start the day without caffeine,
If you can be cheerful, ignoring aches and pains,
If you can resist complaining and boring people with your troubles,
If you can eat your food every day and be grateful for it,
If you can understand when your loved ones are too busy to give you any time,
If you can take criticism and blame without resentment,
If you can conquer tension without medical help,

If you can relax without alcohol,
If you can sleep without the aid of drugs,

Then you're probably the family dog.

Because the immune system is compromised by an allergy attack, it is for this reason I disagree with subjecting Whiskers or Spot to a vaccine until the allergy has been dealt with. Injecting a vaccine into an allergy sufferer may overload an already stressed immune system, often creating a further decline in the pet's health.

I'm unsure if a clinical study has ever been conducted on the relationship between nutrition and pet vaccinations, but if it hasn't, it should be. A vaccination is a planned attack on the immune system. In order to defend itself, the immune system needs to be as robust as possible. Good nutrition is a major support for the immune system. If your pet's food is of poor quality, its immune system cannot be as effective as it should be. On the other had, a nutritious diet will provide a beneficial influence by assisting to keep the immune system operating at peak efficiency. A quality diet will also provide an indirect influence by reducing stresses on digestive organs, in turn reducing stress on the immune system. That's important because you don't want to have a prestressed immune system when a vaccination is administered. While vaccines are intended to prevent harm to the recipient, they are dangerous and can be the cause of harm if the recipient's immune system proves incapable of dealing with them in an efficient manner. There are other negative influences on the immune system, including illness, age, and parasites. Combine any of those with poor nutrition and you have a recipe for disaster, and vaccination disaster is something many pet parents have complained of for years.

For decades pharmaceutical companies and the veterinarian community promoted annual vaccinations against a wide range of diseases impacting cats and dogs. It was a very lucrative practice. Nobody questioned it: it was the right thing to do—so we were told. Sadly, this fear-mongering form of salesmanship is still being implemented today. My daughter recently adopted a friendly little poodle/bichon mix from our local shelter. She was advised his shots were up to date . . . and it was pointedly stated he would require another rabies shot in a year. I guess old habits are difficult to break, as the rabies shot just given him will still be effective in a year's time . . . and beyond. I know that! What I fail to understand is why an animal professional (shelter employee) doesn't know that. For several years there has been an increasing protest against what most pet parents consider a policy of overvaccination of their loved pets. It remains a hot-button topic to this day and likely will remain so for quite some time. (Google *animal vaccinations* and you'll come up with over eighteen million results.)

I don't wish to create the impression that vaccinating our pets is a bad idea. It's actually a good idea; the benefits have never been in doubt. Overvaccinating our pets—like the annual rabies shot promoted by our local shelter—is a bad idea. Most middle-aged or senior people today will recall that incidents of rabies in or near their communities were a common concern years ago. Things have changed. Routine rabies vaccinations commencing in the 1950s has resulted in the dramatic reduction of rabies outbreaks in our pets. A side benefit is that it is now rare for a human to contract rabies from a rabid pet. A downside to the decades-old rabies fear is that many government jurisdictions have laws on the books requiring annual rabies vaccinations; many of these laws remain in place whether valid or not. Other jurisdictions are altering their laws to reflect the availability of three-year rabies vaccines. (That's interesting in that hearsay says the regular rabies vaccine and the three-year rabies vaccine are the same; the latter just costs more.) Other pet diseases, such as distemper and parvovirus in dogs and panleukopenia in cats, were once common, and now, thanks to vaccinations, they appear less frequently today. So yes, vaccines are a good thing.

The players in this vaccination scenario are the pharmaceutical companies, veterinarians, and we paropets. The pharmaceutical companies seem to be holding their ground regarding annual vaccinations: a skeptic may note that their position is, in no small measure, financially motivated. For decades, the veterinarian community was in lockstep with the pharmaceutical manufacturers; like the manufacturers, vets also have a profit motive for frequent vaccinations. It is only the strident voices of a host of unhappy and concerned paropets who have forced this issue to the forefront of pet health care, finally creating a long overdue rift between veterinarians and pharmaceutical companies.

While pharmaceutical companies are standing firm, it's gratifying to observe that a growing number of veterinarians and veterinarian educators are no longer riding the annual vaccination train. It is increasingly recognized within the veterinarian fraternity that reactions to vaccines are more common than previously acknowledged and can be far more serious than once thought. Still, as too many incidences of vaccine reaction are simply shrugged off, thus going unreported, I suspect no one in the animal medical community really has a good idea as to the prevalence of the problem. Thankfully, many in the veterinary community now recognize that a problem exists and have identified a need for vaccine protocol change. In 1998 the American Association of Feline Practitioners dramatically changed the vaccination game by recommending three-year vaccination intervals for most of the core feline vaccines. The floodgates were now open: in no time at all what was good for Whiskers was now considered to be good for Spot. Five years later in 2003, the American Animal Hospital Association Canine Vaccine Task Force recommended three-year booster intervals in adult dogs for parvovirus, distemper virus, adenovirus-2, and parainfluenza virus. Rabies vaccines are also joining this group, as laws dictating their application continue to change.

The issue has not been resolved. How long immunity lasts for each vaccine is still being studied, and there remains a myriad of questions yet to be investigated. Many veterinarians are not accepting the newer recommendations and will vaccinate annually, and animal care workers such as the shelter employee mentioned earlier continue to recommend annual vaccines to unsuspecting adopters. Here's another recent example of overvaccination: only a few months ago a friend took her cat in for its annual checkup. Knowing her indoor cat didn't require a vaccine (having received one the prior year), she was subjected to a combination of guilt tripping and bullying by the vet until she agreed to the vaccine. Next year, she'll be visiting a new veterinarian.

Another problem I have with vaccination protocols is that several vaccines are combined in a single shot . . . a vaccine cocktail (multivalent vaccine). If Whiskers or Spot have a reaction, are they reacting to a single vaccine or the combined dose? We'll likely never know. And the problem can be serious. I worked with a customer whose middle-aged German shepherd had serious health issues, including ongoing hotspots and hair loss. His coat was brittle and dull, and he was somewhat lethargic. We spent the best part of a year experimenting with diet and supplements, slowly making progress. He didn't know why this ailment had befallen his dog, but after several conversations, the suspicion fell on his pet's last vaccination, provided some months earlier. He had returned to his vet a couple of times in the weeks following the vaccination regarding the change in the dog's health. Nothing was found to be obviously wrong with the dog, and the question of a vaccination reaction was never discussed, possibly because the dog had not experienced vaccine-related problems in past years. Regardless, I suspected the vaccine triggered the dog's problems.

Finally, after almost a year, the dog was nearly back to his old self. He was more active, and his coat was shinier, with shedding reduced to normal levels. Success! Then he moved to another town . . . and changed vets. You know where this is going, right! The new vet had the dog in for a physical checkup. Upon discovering it had been over a year since its last vaccination, he/she arbitrarily gave it a new shot. Disaster! The owner was in tears when he came back to me a few days later. The dog was very sick and under observation in the vet's clinic. I don't know the ultimate fate of the dog, as there was nothing further I could do for the owner or his pet. I feared the worst, though.

We should understand that vaccines are preventive medications—not cures. Furthermore, they often require several days before they're effective, as the immune system needs time to ramp up its defenses against the new threat provided by the vaccine. Vaccines work best in healthy, unstressed pets. That being said, it appears to me that many veterinarians who are treating pets for allergy problems don't consider an allergic pet as being unhealthy and will thoughtlessly vaccinate them. I couldn't disagree more with this practice. With a large number of allergy diets available in my store, I deal with many allergic cats and dogs. A pet suffering from allergies is a pet whose immune system is under attack. To vaccinate that pet is to put an additional strain on an already compromised immune system. As I see it, the immune system now has a double burden to deal with and a high risk of a negative result in the offing. I have had so many customers with allergic pets, who, over the years, have reported increased health problems following a vaccination that I now suggest they avoid vaccinations until the allergy issues have been minimized or, preferably, eliminated. I also suggest customers make it very clear to their vet, before a vaccination, that Spot or Whiskers is suffering from an allergy.

For those who are concerned with their pet receiving an annual cocktail of vaccines, some veterinary schools are now suggesting alternative vaccination protocols. Rather than using the combination of vaccines against multiple diseases, they recommend using monovalent vaccines targeting a single disease. One year Spot would be vaccinated against distemper, the next year against canine adenovirus-2, and the third year against parvovirus. Then the cycle would repeat itself, with each disease being readdressed on a three-year rotation. The pet would still receive an annual vaccine, but one more gentle on its immune system. As manufacturers of cat and dog vaccines have not changed their labeling recommending annual vaccinations, each paropet must make an informed choice of when and what to vaccinate. Your veterinarian should help you make the decision.

Warning: Kittens and puppies should not be allowed to associate with other animals in parks, kennels, and doggie daycares until they have completed their initial series of vaccinations, unless your vet advises otherwise. Some vets may approve contact following the second shot.

ALLERGIC PEOPLE

The better I get to know men, the more I find myself loving dogs.

—Charles de Gaulle

While some pets are prone to allergies, some people are allergic to pets. When it comes to cats, my wife is one of those people. (Now you know why we're a dog household.) It's a major problem affecting thousands of people, many of whom would love to have the pleasure of a pet in their lives but cannot due to allergy problems, some of which can be severe.

The main pet-generated culprits for generating human allergies are dander and saliva. It is the proteins found in each that are the allergens. Pet urine is also a cause, although not as common as the other two. While cats and dogs are the usual sources of trouble here, rodents, horses, and indeed any fur-bearing or feathered animal can initiate the development of symptoms. The allergens can be acquired through contact with our skin or inhaled in the air we breathe, making it all but impossible to avoid them. Our body reacts to the allergen by producing histamine, which, in turn, causes hay fever–like or asthmatic symptoms.

While I have no supporting evidence to prove my theory, I suspect that cats, incessant groomers that they are, probably generate more allergens from saliva than skin. Dogs, I'm thinking, are more prone to producing skin dander allergens. This may account for cats, instead of dogs, being considered more responsible for triggering human allergies.

For most people prone to these allergies, like my wife, symptoms are more a nuisance than a problem. Sneezing and red, itchy eyes are about as bad as it gets. The symptoms usually clear up fairly quickly once they have escaped the "pet zone." Often an antihistamine reduces or eliminates the symptoms for them. For others, an allergic reaction may be far more severe, with asthmalike symptoms including chest pain and breathing difficulties. In some cases, anaphylactic reactions may be sufficiently severe as to warrant medical intervention.

Human pet allergy symptoms include:

- Sneezing, coughing
- Red, itchy, watery eyes
- Runny, itchy nose, nasal congestion

Asthmaticlike symptoms include:

- Breathing difficulties, wheezing/whistling when exhaling
- Chest pain
- Sleep deprivation due to other symptoms

An additional symptom is allergic dermatitis. This is normally the result of direct skin contact with an allergen resulting in skin inflammation. Affected skin will become itchy, with rashlike red patches. Some of the symptoms listed above may accompany an allergic dermatitis problem.

Once an allergy sufferer's immune system is compromised, other environmental factors may frequently compound the problem. Air pollution, including tobacco smoke, automotive exhaust fumes, and pollens can all worsen their condition.

Some of the saddest stories I hear in the store are from people who've been forced to give up a beloved pet because a family member has developed an allergy to it. It's definitely a lose/lose situation for everyone, pet included. These events usually happen in a home with children where no one knew in advance that the child was prone to pet allergies. Sometimes they're taken by surprise when the allergic reactions have occurred weeks, even many months, after the pet has been in the home. That happens! Most adults, in comparison, have learned the hard way that they suffer from pet allergies. In the case where pet allergies are known in advance, and if the allergic reaction is not of the severe type, they will often seek out a pet that is less of an offender than others; they want a low-allergy (hypoallergenic) pet.

Contrary to many Internet claims, hypoallergenic pets don't exist. The myth may, in fact, be a child of the Internet. While some individual animals may not trigger allergy reactions as readily as do their peers, experts studying pet allergies claim there's no clinical evidence supporting any breed's hypoallergenic status. The myth seems to be centered on shedding: the less shedding, the lower the incident of allergy reaction, is how the thinking goes. Yes, there are dogs and cats that shed less than their peers; however, less shedding isn't the solution, as hair isn't the allergen. Dander from the skin, along with saliva and urine, are the allergens, as already identified. All skin sheds itself in a constant process of renewal, and all cats and dogs will secrete saliva either through drooling, licking (themselves, you, or other things), or in other manners.

If you wish to have a pet in the home, allergies be damned, there are some suggestions worth considering if the allergy sufferer experiences only a low level of reaction to a pet's presence. These protocols come with no guarantees, and please remember that allergy reactions can worsen over time. Still, if you want to share your home with a pet, these options are better than no options at all. I know they will help. Will they help enough, is the question.

- **Immunotherapy:** A series of shots can be administered that serve to desensitize the person to the allergens generated by the pet. We covered this in the previous chapter in greater detail.

- **Antihistamines:** May be helpful for a short time, but constant, long-term use is not likely a good idea. Immunotherapy is a better solution.
- **Nasal sprays/eye drops:** Prescription sprays and drops may be sufficient to control limited symptoms for some people.
- **Breed of cat:** While I'm unaware of any evidence supporting my view, I suspect that a short-haired cat will do less licking than its long-haired kin, thus generating less saliva. Because cats are dedicated groomers, they may not be an allergy sufferer's best bet for a family pet.
- **Breed of dog:** A smaller dog should cause fewer problems than a larger dog (less skin, less dander). Wiry-haired dogs such as terriers and schnauzers are easier to keep clean than dogs with thick undercoats.
- **Food:** Provide a good-quality food and use an omega-3 supplement, as both will promote healthy skin: healthy skin eliminates excessive dander production.
- **Air purifiers:** There are many products available, some better than others. Prices vary widely. Do your investigating online before you lay out your cash. I'd buy one with a HEPA filter. A good starting point for information is allergybuyersclub.com.
- **Cleanliness:** Bathe the pet often, at least once a month, to wash off any saliva and dander. Between baths, use a damp, clean cloth to wipe down your pet as frequently as you wish, even daily. Vacuum all areas of the home frequently, especially those areas visited by the pet. Use a vacuum cleaner with an HEPA filter. Wash pet bedding frequently.
- **Lifestyle:** Prevent the pet from sleeping on the affected person's bed, or even entering the bedroom.

There you have it. Reducing the impact of pet allergy does take a bit of work, but if it means you can enjoy the wonderful presence of a pet in your home, it's worth it.

CHAPTER 10

Dental Details

As every cat owner knows, nobody owns a cat.

—Ellen Perry

Had I know earlier I was going to write this book, there are many bits and pieces of interesting information I would have retained over the years. Ah, hindsight! An article in a trade journal comes to mind as something I should have saved for today. Instead, we'll have to rely on my unreliable memory for the gist of the article.

Several years ago there was a veterinarian convention in Las Vegas. Staff from a trade magazine greeted arriving vets, asking them to complete a questionnaire. Some questions covered pet dental care, and two of the questions have remained with me in that portion of my brain reserved for "interesting but otherwise useless information" (there should be a television game show for this stuff). One question asked if they (the vets) recommend that pet owners brush their pets' teeth on a daily basis. The positive response was quite high, over 75 percent, if I recall correctly, claiming they provide this advice to clients. The irony was buried in the other question, which asked if they regularly brush their own pets' teeth. The results provide a case of "do what I say versus do what I do," as less than a third admitted they regularly perform this task themselves. Would they be called hypocrites? I'm in no position to criticize the vets on this issue. I, too, recommend my customers clean their pets' teeth daily, or at least frequently, and I, too, am a hypocrite here as I don't brush Taffy's teeth (I do use an oral spray). So, do as I say, not do as I do!

Brushing the teeth of a cat or dog can be a challenge, especially if you're starting the process with an older pet. If they aren't accustomed to it, be very, very patient. Otherwise, you'll likely have a war on your hands and create a situation impossible to rectify later. It's always easiest to implement regular brushing with puppies and kittens—the younger, the better. Even then you will want to exercise great patience, commencing with small steps eventually leading to a proper brushing. There are additional advantages to this process other than simply keeping the teeth clean. While brushing, you have an opportunity to inspect the teeth and gums for any signs of problems, such as gum lesions or tooth chipping, which might warrant a vet examination. There are other problems to look for, and we'll discuss them in a moment.

Does this regular tooth-brushing regimen seem like a lot of work for nothing? The American Veterinary Medical Association estimates that more than 80 percent of dogs and 70 percent of cats over three years of age have significant dental disease. Other veterinary organizations put those numbers even higher. If you want your pet to fit in with the healthy group, you are not wasting your time by providing oral care. Consider it preventive maintenance, implemented for all the same reasons you brush your own teeth. If you're motivated by a financial incentive, ask your vet about the cost of having Whiskers's or Spot's teeth cleaned—that procedure is anything but cheap!

Oral care products are available from any pet supply retailer and are usually inexpensive. There are two types of toothbrushes: one that looks like a smaller version of your toothbrush, and one called a finger brush. The former should have a fairly soft bristle (a baby toothbrush can be substituted). The latter (finger brush) is made of rubber in a tubelike form that slides on your finger and has rubber bristles on the end for the scrubbing action. Toothpaste comes in both feline and canine versions (or a combo) and usually has a meaty flavor to encourage a favorable reception. Most pet toothpastes are enzymatic; they work by leaving enzymes in the mouth that target and help destroy plaque and tartar buildups. There are other products available that I'll cover shortly.

Warning: Never use human toothpaste on your pet. Chemicals in human products can be detrimental to your pet's health if swallowed. Keep in mind that when we brush our teeth, we normally

spit out the toothpaste and rinse thoroughly when finished. Whiskers and Spot aren't good at spitting or rinsing, and they will ingest the toothpaste instead.

For pet owners about to start on the adventure of pet oral care, I would suggest, before you lay out any money on dental supplies, that you see if you can get your finger safely into your pet's mouth. It's easier for dogs, as you can get them to open up with a bit of peanut butter or ketchup on the tip of a finger. With cats, a bit of their favorite canned food or yogurt might do the trick. First, treat your fingertip and let them lick it off two or three times. Do that for a day or two. Next, place your treated finger right in their mouth, but only for a second or two. Continue this process over a period of days   and several times a day—gradually keeping your finger in their mouth for longer and longer periods.

However, don't do your happy dance just yet, as you haven't crossed the finish line. If the process seems to be working (as in you've retained all of your fingers), visit your favorite pet supply store and obtain some suitable oral care products. Now that you have some toothpaste, begin switching from your original inducement to the toothpaste to allow them an opportunity to adjust to the new flavor. If they balk at the toothpaste, mix a bit of it with whatever tasty bribe you were originally using.

Say, did I mention patience?

Once they're okay with the toothpaste, put lots of it on their toothbrush and start the slow process all over. It should go faster now, as they're only adjusting to the feel of the brush. As they become accustomed to that, try a gentle scrub for a few seconds, gradually building the time up until you can actually brush their teeth.

Congratulations! You've made it! There should be a certificate awarded to those who reach this noble goal.

Note: For beginners interested in commencing pet oral care, an excellent online video is provided by the American Veterinary Medical Association (avma.org). This short video covers the techniques required, with demonstrations using both cats and dogs. I recommend watching this video prior to implementing your pet's oral care program.

With the prevalence of dental disease in our pet population, it's probably safe to assume that, after two years of age, disease is likely present in varying degrees depending on differing factors such as lifestyle and diet. Common indicators of oral problems include:

- Bad breath
- Swollen, bleeding gums
- Discolored teeth
- Plaque buildup
- Appetite loss
- Discomfort while eating
- Pawing and rubbing the face
- Drooling

There are several types of oral disease found in our cats and dogs. Some will require veterinary care, while others may be eliminated or reduced in severity through proper care, including regular brushing and inspection. Common problems are those such as the following:

Feline ondoclastic resorptive lesions: These are not normally associated with younger cats. Ondoclast cells commence resorbing the tooth, creating a very painful condition for Whiskers. The cause is unknown and there is no cure, but proper dental health and a strong immune system supported with good nutrition may slow the disease's progression and lessen its impact on your cat. This is the second most common oral disease in our felines.

Abnormal wear: This condition results in excessive wear patterns on teeth. It often appears in pets with very long jaws, such as greyhounds and collies, or those with short jaws such as pugs, but it may occur with any pet, especially those who aggressively chew hard toys or abrasive objects. Did you know that the nylon fuzz on a tennis ball is abrasive and can harm the teeth of any dog constantly chewing it?

Gingivitis: This is caused by tartar buildup on the teeth close to the gum line. The gums can become sore and inflamed, eventually shrinking and receding and exposing more tooth surface to tartar buildup. Untreated, the infection can worsen, creating a great deal of pain for your pet. The disease can often be reversed with the removal of accumulated tartar and the implementation of proper oral care.

Periodontal disease: This is the most common oral disease for both cats and dogs. An infection, deep in the gums, attacks the periodontal membrane, which then loses its attachment to the root of the tooth, resulting in a loose tooth that often falls out (pyorrhea). Eating becomes so painful your pet may start to lose weight. Unchecked, the disease will attack other teeth. These anaerobic bacteria require sugar to survive and thrive. Proper oral hygiene to reduce plaque buildup and oral bacteria is the best defense, along with a sugar-free diet and treats.

Toothache and tooth decay: These problems can be difficult to identify. If your pet is frequently pawing or rubbing his or her face, or is crying without apparent cause, it's probably time to have the vet check for causes that are not obvious during normal oral inspections.

Tooth fractures: Mostly a problem for Spot. Many dogs love to chew objects; often, the harder, the better. I have customers who are frustrated because a new chew toy was demolished within days, and sometimes even within hours. I've had toys described as "indestructible" by the manufacturer end up trashed in no time at all. Frequently, these customers will look for the hardest, most durable chew toy they can find, hoping to take something home that will last long enough for them to get their money's worth. While I understand their frustration, I also recognize that the harder the toy the greater the wear on their dog's teeth, and the greater the risk of having a tooth fracture as a result of the hard chew. I realize these paropets are between a rock and a hard place here, but a really, really hard chew toy may not be in the best interest of their dog's dental health. For puppies still retaining their baby teeth, I never suggest hard chew toys because of the danger of damage to those young teeth and the potential to create problems when adult teeth emerge later. Other causes of fractured teeth are games such as Frisbee or the use of a fairly hard rubber or plastic ball for catching, especially if catching in the air when the combined velocity of both toy and dog is quite high.

Along with regular oral care such as brushing, there are other procedures you can implement to help maintain a healthy mouth for Spot and Whiskers. Generally speaking, these products are helpful for that pet that simply won't—under any circumstance—let you work in its mouth.

Nutrition: Select nutritious foods that will support your pet's immune system, enabling it to fight all disease, including oral types. The foods should be of the low-starch varieties (no corn, wheat, rice) and contain no added sugar sources. This also applies to all treats, as they will often contain sugar sources added to be attractive to your pet's taste buds. Read the ingredients on the package before making your purchase.

Drinking water additives: These are products that you add to your pet's drinking water to help combat plaque and tartar. They can be effective but are not a quick fix, in that the benefit they provide is cumulative, with results appearing over time.

Tip: When using drinking water additives, it can be a nuisance mixing the small amount required into Whiskers's or Spot's water bowl every time a refill is required. Instead, premix it into a large water jug or empty plastic beverage (soda pop or juice) bottle and keep that in the refrigerator, ready for use at any time.

Oral sprays: Like other oral care additives, these products are not a quick fix and usually produce their best results if used consistently over time. Easy to use, they normally require a quick spray into the mouth once or twice daily. Most are a combination of herbal extracts and other ingredients designed to stimulate the pet's natural enzymatic defenses against tartar and plaque. Some, like Leba III (lebalab.com), are quite expensive; however, a small bottle will usually last up to nine months (I tell customers it's expensive to buy but, over eight or nine months, inexpensive to use). As pricey as some of these products may be, they're a lot less expensive than having your pet's teeth cleaned at your veterinary clinic. There are less expensive options, such as those provided by PetzLife (petzlife.com), which also seem to work well.

Oral gels: These work much like the sprays except they're in gel form. You apply the gel directly to the teeth and let the product go to work. Gels are normally available in pet-pleasing flavors. The application only takes a couple of seconds, which should not deter even the most attention-deficit cat or dog.

Note: Instructions for both sprays and gels often state that they should not be applied within thirty minutes before or after a meal. The reason for this is that you want the ingredients to linger in the mouth rather than being absorbed by food and water and quickly swallowed. It's probably wise to remove their water bowl for the before/after the thirty-minute period.

If you are able to brush your pet's teeth, you may still wish to use an oral spray, gel, or drinking water additive as they will provide additional support toward maintaining good oral care. For pets that won't tolerate a daily brushing, the use of these products daily, followed by a once- or twice-weekly brushing, will likely result in a beneficial outcome. Whatever you do, it's better than doing nothing.

There are also a variety of dental treats for both cats and dogs that will help keep teeth clean. Some of these use questionable ingredients such as propylene glycol, so be sure to review the ingredient list prior to purchasing. For dogs, there is a wide assortment of dental chew toys on the market. Your pet supply retailer will have several to select from, including rawhide chews, which can also be beneficial.

Note: Rawhide chews can be dangerous. If a large piece of rawhide is swallowed, it can obstruct the bowel. The rawhide I prefer dogs to use is referred to as "pressed rawhide"; pressed rawhide is less likely to provide a large, dangerous piece. This type of treat is made from rawhide compressed under high pressure into various shapes (like a bone, for example). While more expensive than rawhide strips, it will last much longer. All rawhide should be used only under supervision. Once chewed down to a size that can be swallowed, it should be discarded.

In an earlier chapter I mentioned that I suspect starchy, grain-rich diets as being significant contributors to dental problems in today's pet population. The problem with starch is its stickiness, allowing it to coat teeth and become a food supply for the bacteria that are detrimental to good oral health. Unlike human saliva, which generates the amylase enzyme required to convert starch to sugar, our pets' saliva is unequipped for this task. Little by little, the excessive starch found in these diets assists in creating a deteriorating dental condition. It's worth a bit of redundancy here to again point out that products containing sugar as an ingredient compound your pet's dental problems. For this reason, I suggest feeding good-quality diets in which starchy grains are not dominating the ingredient list and sugars have not been included in the formula. The same suggestions apply to treats.

Proponents of raw diets often boast how these diets support cleaner teeth in both cats and dogs. There is likely some truth to these claims, as raw foods, like other grain-free diets, are lacking in the starches so prevalent in grain-rich foods. However, comparisons made to the cleanliness of teeth in wild canines and felines versus domesticated pets can be misleading; most of the wild relatives don't enjoy the long lifespans available to our pets (for example, gray wolves' life spans average six to eight years), therefore, their teeth have much less opportunity to develop serious age-related dental problems.

Some canine breeds seem to be more prone to dental problems than do others. Adult dogs have forty-two teeth. Generally speaking, smaller breeds such as Yorkshire terriers, Maltese, pugs, Papillons, and shih tzus, with their smaller jaws, seem to have more dental issues than their larger cousins, in part due to the number of teeth that must be squeezed into the jaws.

CHAPTER 11

Urinary Disorders

Cats seem to go on the principle that it never does any harm to ask for what you want.

—Joseph Wood Krutch

Too many cat owners have become familiar with feline urinary disorders, and many of them could write this chapter themselves based on their experiences dealing with the problem. However, dog owners need not skip this section, as many canines also are victims of urinary problems. For both cat and dog, here are the main symptoms of a urinary malady:

- Increase in the frequency of urination
- Urinating in unusual places (common with cats)
- Strong ammonia smell in the urine
- Reduced urine output
- Dribbling urine

- Blood in the urine
- Obvious pain/discomfort when urinating (yowls/yelps)
- Inability to urinate

The first five points above should be considered warning flags demanding your close attention. If symptoms worsen or continue for too long, an examination by your vet is strongly advised. The three last points warrant immediate attention from a veterinarian, as inattention can lead to death. One of the following is likely the cause of the symptoms listed above:

Cystitis: This bladder inflammation is caused by a bacterial infection in dogs, and it is the most common source of canine urinary problems. Bacterial infections are rarely the cause of urinary problems in cats; when feline cystitis does occur, it will often be resolved without medical intervention. Instead, felines are more prone to problems created by the formation of urinary stones that can block the urethra, a more rare cause in dogs. The bacterial action causing cystitis can happen on its own, but there can be other triggers such as bladder stones or tumors. Treatment involves administering antibiotics to fight the infection and surgery if stones or polyps must be removed.

Urinary stones: There are two types of stones commonly seen: calcium oxalate and struvite. Because of the opposing urine pH conditions required for the development of each stone variety, animals with calcium oxalate stones tend not to have struvites, and vice versa.

Note: The pH of a liquid symbolizes the acidity or alkalinity. Seven is neutral—any value lower than seven is acidic (low pH), and higher is alkaline (high pH). A slightly acidic urine pH of six to 6.6 is ideal for most pets.

Calcium oxalate stones: All urine contains a small amount of calcium oxalate, which only becomes problematic when levels increase. These stones are usually associated with low magnesium and a high level of acid and calcium in the urine. Once formed, oxalate stones cannot be eliminated with a change in diet and will not dissolve in urine. The urinary system can be flushed to eliminate those stones small enough to pass through the urethra, but larger stones can only be removed surgically.

Dog or cat, most victims are males, as males have a narrower urethra than females. Cats over five years of age are at greatest risk, as are indoor cats. There appears to be a hereditary influence for this stone formation; Dalmatians, for example, are far more prone to the disease than other dogs, as are Burmese and Himalayan cats. Potential oxalate stone development is addressed with veterinarian preventative diets for those pets at risk of developing them. These diets rely on reduced protein levels and added potassium citrate to alter urine pH. As most of these diets are heavily grain based, their use may be the lesser of two evils where your pet's nutrition is concerned.

While these stones were uncommon in felines two or three decades ago, commercial cat foods may be unintentionally contributing to the increased frequency of the formation of calcium oxalate stones. When high-magnesium and low urine pH levels (acidic) were identified by researchers as the main cause in the rise of feline struvite problems, pet food manufactures began reducing the amount of magnesium in their diets while at the same time adding urine acidifiers. The change successfully reduced the incidence of cats suffering from struvites, which is a good thing. Unfortunately, a decrease in struvite problems directly coincided with an increase in the number of cats suffering from oxalate stones as a result of this well-intentioned but misguided urine tampering. Today, oxalate stones may account for up to a half of all feline urinary stone problems.

Struvite stones: These stones are a common feline problem. While not as prevalent in dogs, the greater majority of canine victims are females. Some studies have identified magnesium as being the principal cause of struvite uroliths, along with a high urine pH level (alkaline). Other studies suggest that pH levels may be the dominant factor in their formation. Regardless of clinical results, it's obvious that an alkaline urine and excessive magnesium provides a one-two punch leading to the formation of these uroliths. Acidic urine helps to dissolve these stones as well as preventing their formation in the first place.

Veterinarian "dissolution diets" are often provided for clearing up struvite stones. These diets use ammonium chloride and methionine to generate the highly acidic urine required to dissolve struvite crystals. Such diets are intended for short-term use only, up to three months. When symptoms have cleared, gradually transition your pet to a suitable diet for long-term use. Dissolution diets should not be used with kittens, pregnant/nursing queens, or pets with high blood pressure or kidney disease.

Obviously, by increasing/decreasing acidifiers and magnesium levels in food, it is clear that food can play an important role in your pet's urinary health. One of the food ingredients now often included in better-quality cat foods (and some dog foods) is cranberry. Cranberries have a long association with urinary health in humans as a preventative measure against urinary problems, and it seems the benefits these berries provide may also be helpful to our pets, although a representative of the Cranberry Institute advised me that they are unaware of any research supporting such claims for pets. That being said, I believe we can optimistically expect that cranberry products will provide similar urinary health benefits for Whiskers and Spot as they do for us. I leave it to the Cranberry Institute (cranberryinstitute.org) to explain cranberry's healthy impact: "Cranberries contain proanthocyanidins (PACs), which inhibit the fimbrial adhesion of bacteria, including *Escherichia coli*, to the urinary tract epithelium and hence the subsequent reproduction required for infection. It is these unique compounds that are pivotal in the prevention of UTI (urinary tract infection) rather than the acidification of the urine as was previously hypothesized."

When dealing with urinary issues, in addition to veterinarian instructions, I often recommend that paropets get some cranberry into their four-footers. The easiest way is to find a pet food that incorporates cranberry in its ingredient list, common now in better-quality cat foods. Additionally, add some juice to their water. Dogs may love it, but cats may be slower to accept the juice. Start with a few drops and slowly increase the amount over several days. Another option is to obtain a powdered cranberry supplement from a pet food supplier, pharmacy, or health food store and incorporate it into their regular diet. The supplement or juice, used daily, may be a beneficial dietary aid in preventing future urinary issues, or may reduce the severity of symptoms for those pets prone to chronic urinary infections. In addition to cranberry, a good-quality fish oil supplement can be beneficial. This oil will provide vitamins A and D, both contributors to urinary health, along with the other benefits associated with omega-3 fatty acids.

Diet, as mentioned, can play an important role in urinary health. For a pet suffering from urinary difficulties, I recommend evaluating the food it was eating when the problem occurred. I'd be concerned with any food that is grain rich, along with high-fiber diets such as feline hairball formulas; excessive fiber tends to direct water through the bowel, reducing the amount of liquid needed for an appropriate urine pH, as well as for properly flushing the urinary tract. Grain-rich diets tend not to be as dense as meat-rich diets, thus requiring your pet to eat more food for adequate nutrition. Additional food requires additional water for stool formation, thereby reducing the water available for flushing the urinary tract.

As discussed in an earlier chapter, not all pets drink sufficient water throughout the day, an important factor that doesn't seem to attract as much attention as it should. I always recommend paropets monitor their pet's water intake for a few days to determine if sufficient water is being ingested and to take appropriate measures to increase it if required. An increase in water consumption alone may be sufficient to prevent the onset or recurrence of some urinary problems. Some methods of getting additional water into our pets are as follows:

- Add water or broth to kibble, dehydrated, or freeze-dried foods, and let it soak in.
- Add some canned food to the meal, or switch to canned foods.
- Switch to frozen diets, baked or raw; both possess more water than dry kibble.

Here are some other contributors to urinary problems. Most are easily altered lifestyle changes; a change now may head off future vet bills.

- Free-feeding may create urinary tract issues as pets allowed to nibble all day may generate urine with an elevated pH, leading to the formation of struvite crystals.
- Exercise is important. Sedentary and overweight pets are more prone to urinary problems. All pets will benefit from some daily activity in the form of walks and play.
- Indoor cats frequently holding urine while waiting for a clean litter box may develop stones.
- Dogs waiting for long periods to be let out to urinate may develop stones.
- A sudden diet change may cause urinary issues, especially in pets unused to a change in their food. The sudden diet change may create a change in urine pH, resulting in a problem.

Regardless of the steps you take, urinary problems may show up again in months or years, as some have a high rate of recurrence. However, don't throw in the towel, as the word *may* is operative here. An appropriate diet, sufficient water intake, lifestyle changes, and suitable supplements *may*—alone or in combination   keep urinary problems at bay for the remainder of your pet's life.

As noted in this chapter, using diet to tamper with our pets' urinary pH levels has, in some instances, led to widespread urinary health issues.

There are various dietary supplements on the market designed to reduce the severity of canine urine burns on lawns and shrubs. I've long assumed that, in order to benefit your lawn, these products need to alter Spot's urine pH. While good for lawns, this alteration may not be good for Spot or your pocketbook if a urinary health problem results. When I've questioned manufacturers regarding this, they get a bit dodgy. I refuse to sell their products, as they've failed to convince me they're safe for Spot, and I suggest you also be cautious.

CHAPTER 12

The Scoop on Poop

If your dog is fat, you aren't getting enough exercise!

—Anonymous

For whatever reason, pet poop is a major topic of conversation with paropets. The bad news is that there are as many opinions on poop as there are pet parents. Some of those opinions are valid; others aren't worth the time it takes to pick them up and throw them out.

One of the subjects arising time and again is that of dogs out for a walk. Customers will come in to the store thinking there's something wrong with their dog's bowel movements (BMs) because Spot poops more than once during the walk. The first movement is usually firm, but the second often quite soft. What's wrong with Spot?

Nothing is wrong with your dog. Taffy usually has two BMs in the first twenty minutes of each walk. The second is always softer than the first. On those trips when she has a third BM, I refuse to describe its consistency. Yuck! Most dogs love going for a walk or romp. They get excited. The excitement—plus the exercise—triggers follow-up BMs. The first BM, already positioned to vacate the premises, is normally firm. The next, being hurried along by circumstances, is almost always softer. It's natural. Quit worrying about it. There's nothing wrong with your pet's bowels, or their diet.

Stool firmness is another popular topic. Too many cat and dog owners are of the opinion their pets' stools should have the firmness of a kiln-baked brick. It always shocks me when I hear this. Come on, folks! I realize rock-hard feces are more convenient for scooping or picking up, but still! It's not like you're going to slingshot the feces into neighbors' yards three or four houses away, is it? I suspect if your own stools came out rock hard, you'd be heading for the prunes or bran flakes at a fast trot. Exceptionally firm stools are probably not good for your pet and may indicate insufficient liquid consumption. Conversely, stools that are always voluminous and soft might also be problematic. In addition to making yard cleanup more difficult, very soft stools may not be helping anal glands express themselves and may also indicate either overfeeding and/or feeding an overly fibrous food such as a grain-rich diet. A normal stool should be firm but not hard, and certainly not sloppy soft (walks aside as previously mentioned). In fact, they should be similar to what you consider to be a good stool for yourself.

Constipation constantly pops up in pet poop conversations (can you say that line ten times quickly?). Diet can be one cause of constipation; exercise, or its lack, another part of the problem. A third factor, which many people seem unaware of, veterinarians included, is liquid intake. Taffy is a water drinker. She drinks a lot of water throughout the day. This is common for her (no, she's not diabetic). In conversations with pet owners complaining of ongoing pet constipation, I came to realize that not all cats and dogs are good at imbibing sufficient water throughout the day. Further, when talking to pet owners who have taken their pet to a vet regarding constipation issues, I note vets often fail to inquire about the pet's liquid intake (the topic comes up in relation to urinary problems, but not for constipation). While constipation impacts both felines and canines, it seems our cats suffer more from this problem than dogs. I can't tell you why this is, just that, anecdotally, it appears to be the case.

The problem for cats and smaller dogs drinking insufficient water is an increased risk of dehydration due to their smaller stature. It's still a serious problem for larger animals, but size mitigates the level of concern . . . a little. Dehydration leads to constipation. If your pet is frequently constipated, I suggest you commence monitoring its water intake, as this could be the problem. We've all heard the expression "you can lead a horse to water but you can't make it drink." Well, the same is true for the cat and dog that fails to imbibe sufficient water throughout the day. How do you make that pet drink more? It can be a challenge. Here are some suggestions.

Flowing water might be the answer. I had a customer with a cat that would drink from a dripping tap rather than from his water bowl; he seemed to prefer moving water that, for whatever reason, seems to trigger drinking instincts in many of our pets, particularly cats. I suspect there's some ancestral memory of drinking from wilderness streams at play here, but hey, I'm guessing. There are electronic water dishes available that constantly circulate water. While these electronic water bowls aren't cheap, they're cheaper than regular visits to the vet to clean up a chronic constipation problem. Before you try the electronic bowl, try adding a bit of low-salt chicken or beef broth to your pet's water bowl. Sometimes just a bit of flavor will do the trick. You probably don't need to add much broth to generate interest.

Replacing kibble in all or part with wet food will help. This can be canned food or raw/baked/dehydrated (if rehydrated) diets. Another option is to simply add some water or broth to their regular kibble food. Give the kibble a few minutes in which to absorb the liquid, and then feed it to the pet. However you manage it, it's imperative to get sufficient liquid into your cat or dog on a daily basis.

Introducing fiber into your pet's diet will also help alleviate constipation. Fiber works hand-in-hand with water by absorbing and holding the water in the bowel. Retaining water in the bowel provides a double benefit in that the water will soften the stool as well as help lubricate the bowel. For cats, it can be somewhat challenging to get sufficient fiber into them. Mixing a bit of dietary fiber such as psyllium (Metamucil or its no-name equivalents) into canned or other wet food, or yogurt, cottage cheese, and sour cream, will often do the trick. For dogs, psyllium also works, as do bran flakes, which most dogs love. (Ensure it's not a sugary cereal or raisin bran flakes, as they don't need sugar and raisins are toxic to dogs.) Also, it is best not to use flavored psyllium: the flavoring is often orange citrus that might turn off a dog, and you can be assured it will likely be refused by your cat.

When adding in fiber to the diet, it's important to strike the correct balance between too much and too little. If too little, you won't solve the problem; if too much, you may pull excess water into the bowel, leaving insufficient water available for good urinary health.

Note: While milk may work for some pets as an incentive to take in more liquid, some caution is needed. First, unlike a majority of

**people, most cats and dogs are lactose intolerant. If you're buy-
ing milk to increase a pet's liquid intake, only buy the lactose-free
products from your supermarket. Second, water down the milk as
much as possible because milk contains solids: your pet needs the
water, not the solids.**

No discussion of pets and their poop can be complete without talking
about constipation's evil twin, diarrhea.

There are many causes of diarrhea; some are dangerous gastrointestinal issues that can only be dealt with through a veterinarian's expert
care. Serious or prolonged bouts of diarrhea definitely warrant a speedy
trip to your veterinarian, even super speedy if you identify blood in the
feces. Often, if not a serious bout, it was caused by ingesting something,
such as overfeeding; eating something too rich or too fatty; eating things
while out for a walk (Taffy's specialty); ingesting toxic foods such as
chocolate; eating overly generous amounts of leftovers; or aggressively
changing to a new diet. If the problem is not serious enough for your
vet's attention, there are several easily administered home remedies that
are usually quite effective at bringing the problem to a halt.

Surprisingly, most solutions for diarrhea again involve the use of
fiber—one of the cures for constipation, as just discussed. Fiber for
both diarrhea and constipation, you ask? Yes indeed! Here's how fiber
works. As mentioned for constipation, fiber holds water in the bowel,
which assists in softening the stool and lubricating the bowel. The key
to remember here is *holds water*. Clearly, in cases of diarrhea, in order
to flush the bowel of something deemed undesirable, the body has
directed an excessive amount of water to the bowel to cleanse it of the
irritant. As fiber holds water, it will help by absorbing much of the excessive water now being supplied by the body. The stools may be softer
than normal for a bit, but the watery mess will soon clear up, enabling
the bowel and Spot or Whiskers to return to normal much faster than
they might have otherwise. An additional benefit of increasing the fiber
is that it may help bind whatever it is the body considers undesirable,
thus hastening the bowel's cleansing process.

For cats (I'm being redundant here), the simplest way for getting
them to ingest some fiber is to sneak something such as psyllium into
anything they'll happily eat: this could be a wet or canned food, or a

bit of yogurt, cottage cheese, or sour cream. Again, psyllium works for dogs, as do bran flakes. Also for dogs, other household foods will assist in achieving beneficial results. Many customers will cook a bit of white rice or peel and microwave a potato and feed that to their dog. The size of the potato should be relative to the size of your dog . . . big dog, big potato; small dog, small potato. A meal or two of rice or potato should reel the back end into line.

Warning: Any period of extended or recurring constipation or diarrhea warrants a visit to your vet for a checkup to determine the cause of the problem.

I'm not a fan of hairball kibble for felines. Most hairball kibble foods I have seen are high-fiber diets; the additional fiber provided is being used to help move ingested hair through the stomach and bowel. Recall that AAFCO regulations only require feeding trials of twenty-six weeks. My concern is that long-term use of a high-fiber diet may be detrimental to Whiskers's health. Specifically, with fiber's ability to hold water in the bowel, I'm concerned that insufficient water is available to support good urinary tract health. Urinary problems can be a major health issue, as many cat owners can testify, particularly with males, whose urinary tracts are much narrower than that of females. Male or female, the urinary tract requires an adequate supply of water to keep their systems appropriately flushed. Long-term use of excessive fiber may well be detrimental to good urinary health in cats.

Instead of hairball diets, I suggest using the hairball treatment available from any pet supply retailer. These products are similar to a small tube of toothpaste. The content is a mild laxative, flavored to appeal to cats . . . well, most cats. Some, of course, don't know what's good for them. If Whiskers refuses to lick it off your finger, lightly press it into the top of a front paw firmly enough so that it can't be flicked off. Whiskers will do the rest. It can also be mixed in with something the cat likes to eat, such as canned food or a small amount of yogurt. If you believe your cat has a hairball, use the hairball treatment every other day for a week or until the hairball has passed. After that, a maintenance application once a week should suffice for most short-haired cats, and twice weekly for long-haired cats.

Cats that shed hair excessively are more prone to hairballs than cats with normal shedding. I have found that excessive shedding is frequently a result of an inferior diet. If your cat—or dog—is shedding too much, upgrade the quality of its food. You can also add an omega-3 supplement to their diet, but before implementing that a simple improvement in the quality of their diet will often solve the problem.

Tip: As hairball medication for cats is a mild laxative, it can be used to assist a pet with a constipation problem.

One of the most unlovable aspects of dog ownership is that of owning a poop-eating dog. Coprophagia is the correct term, but who uses words like that? It's almost enough to turn a dog lover into a cat lover, as cats, being superior creatures (who can disagree?), don't indulge in this disgusting habit. (If they do, they apparently do it in secret.)

No, it seems to be that it's only our dogs that consider poop to be an edible delicacy. It wouldn't be so bad if your dog—having feasted on a feces—didn't think you were in immediate need of canine affection (why do dogs assume this?). A big, wet, dog kiss is NOT what you're interested in then . . . or later (until you've successfully blocked the poop-eating event from your memory).

I'm not sure why some dogs eat feces. Theories abound! I recall, as a child, watching dogs run out from neighboring houses to gobble freshly dropped manure donated by the horse pulling the milk wagon (yes, I'm that old). Later, I read that wolves, coyotes, and wild dogs will eat feces dropped by various herbivores, and that these feces are a terrific source of digestive enzymes that benefit the carnivores (rather like humans ingesting probiotics and digestive enzymes, I suppose). Taffy, for one, does a good job of cleaning up the small mounds of rabbit poop that frequently appear in my yard. It's still disgusting, but for those animals, it makes sense if they're receiving an enzyme or vitamin benefit.

Generally speaking, it isn't particularly dangerous for dogs to eat their own feces, and only marginally dangerous to those eating the feces of other dogs. In households with both a cat and dog, the dog will sometimes develop a taste for the cat's feces. This is a danger if the dog is retrieving cat feces from clumping clay litter, as too much clumping litter, with its liquid-binding properties, may result in a serious health issue if swallowed. Removing ingested clumping litter is difficult, and surgery is risky because the litter will extend throughout the intestine. Another danger results from acquiring intestinal parasites after eating infested cat or dog feces; you might wish to have a poop-eating dog checked regularly for parasites. A pancreatic disorder (pancreatic insufficiency) may also be creating the problem. For these reasons, any dog eating feces should quickly receive a checkup from a veterinarian, particularly if the behavior is newly acquired.

Breaking this behavior can take some effort, ingenuity, and patience. Even though most puppies will grow out of the habit, efforts should be made to discourage the practice as soon as possible; you don't want the habit to continue for even one day longer than needed. The first step is to eliminate the snack source. If the cat's poop is the target, this means ensuring that the dog has no access to the cat's litter box. Position the litter tray where the dog can't reach it, use a covered litter box, barricade the litter behind a baby gate, or anything else you can think of that will keep the litter and the dog apart.

For dogs eating their own poop, your best defense is to beat them to the source; pick it up before they can access it. While this requires some vigilance and dedication on your part, it is probably your best course of action. Another method of discouraging Spot from snacking is to beat him to the stool and generously douse it with the hottest hot sauce or cayenne pepper you can find. This also takes some effort on your part, but it has proven to be effective for many dogs. (Others have learned to enjoy the hot sauce and start to crave TexMex.) You have to get all the feces in the yard, though, as Spot's nose is easily able to discriminate between booby-trapped stools and those safe to chow down on.

If your dog is tempted by the leftovers provided by other dogs, you'll need to be vigilant on walks, ensuring Spot cannot access any feces other dog owners, in their ignorance, have failed to harvest. Even having him wear a muzzle when wandering in the backyard, or while on walks, will help prevent unwanted feces consumption.

Note: Scolding, yelling, or punishing your dog is just about the worst thing you can do. In addition to not providing the results you wish, it may in fact make matters worse.

Another option is changing Spot's diet. If you're using a poor-quality, grain-rich food, try a better diet, or switch from a kibble to a baked food. Your dog may simply be trying to obtain more nutrition than that provided by its present diet. Also, if there's no concern for being overweight, try increasing the dog's food by about 25 percent; he may be eating feces because he's hungry. Still with food, try dividing the dog's daily food ration up into smaller, more frequent servings; Spot still gets the same amount of food, but it's provided in four or more servings during the day rather than two.

Digestive enzymes may prove beneficial by improving the dog's ability to digest its food, thus acquiring more nutrition from each meal. Most pet food retailers should be able to provide suitable enzyme products. Your trainer and veterinarian may provide tips to eliminate this undesirable behavior. Also, your veterinarian and pet supply store may have supplements that are designed to make the stool less palatable. Personally, I have found these items to be ineffective and no longer sell them, but if all else fails, they're worth a try.

Stool eating is a behavior that is best halted as soon as possible. Then, when Spot feels that you need a big wet kiss, you can welcome the love.

A LETTER ABOUT LITTER

> All of the animals except for man know that the principle business
> of life is to enjoy it.
>
> —Samuel Butler

The need for indoor feline toilet facilities is a direct result of responsible cat owners no longer allowing their pets to roam—that's the first part of the good news. The second part of the good news is that we humans were smart enough to design an indoor toilet facility for our felines, and cats were smart enough to figure out how to use it; thus, litter and a litter box came into being. Sometimes the best ideas are the simplest ones.

The world of cat litter has changed significantly over the years. First to arrive on the scene was dried clay litter. The product was inexpensive and did a good job of absorbing liquid, and a scoop quickly got rid of the feces. This clay wasn't too great at odor control, though, so its next evolutionary step was the addition of fragrance or baking soda to mask odors. You use only a small amount of this litter at a time, about one-inch deep in the tray, but it is necessary to completely replace the litter frequently, sometimes daily. These litters are dusty and track.

Next to arrive were the clumping clay litters. The clumping results from the use of bentonite clay that captures the urine before it can sink to the bottom of the tray and holds it in a clump. In order to work properly, you need to use three to four inches of litter in the tray. This makes it easier to scoop up both the urine clumps along with the feces. Clumping litter doesn't have to be replaced as often as clay litter, only requiring the addition of a bit more litter to replace that lost to scooping. For odor control, fragrance and baking soda are often added to these products, especially for multicat formulas. Over time, clumping litter has all but forced its nonclumping predecessor into extinction. Clumping litter, being finer, is even dustier than regular clay litter.

Tip: If you find clumps are sticking to the sides and bottom of the tray, after you empty and clean the tray, spray the sides and bottom with a light mist of cooking oil spray before adding the new litter.

Both of the above litters are notorious for tracking (bits of litter on the floor in a trail from the litter box). These bits stick to the cat's feet as it leaves the litter box and fall off as Whiskers walks around the house. If you're not wearing slippers, the bits will soon stick to your feet.

Tip: You can significantly reduce litter tracking by purchasing an inexpensive coco fiber mat (a door mat) and placing it outside of the litter box, forcing the cat to walk across it as it leaves the box. Make sure you buy a mat with a coarse, toothbrush-style surface versus a smooth surface. The larger the mat you have space for, the more litter you'll capture before it tracks to the rest of the house.

Clay litters have dominated the market for decades, and clumping clay litter continues to be the product used in most homes. However, in recent years, some new arrivals have appeared on retailers' shelves.

Most of the new players are biodegradable, and some are clumpable, compostable, and can be safely flushed down the toilet. The latter feature is important because it is estimated that each year over two million tons of cat litter, or approximately one hundred thousand truckloads, ends up in landfills in the United States alone (www.en.wikipedia .org/wiki/litter_box). (You are forced to wonder who worked out that statistic.)

These new litters are made from a variety of sources, the most common being:

- Pine pellets, both coarse (nonclumping) and finely ground (clumping)
- Wheat
- Ground corn
- Recycled paper
- Silicate crystals (nonclumping)
- Ground walnut shells

Some of these litters provide superior odor control without the addition of fragrances or baking soda, which is a benefit as cats may object to the added fragrances. Most are dust free, or nearly so, in comparison to clay litters. These litters may be more expensive to purchase initially, but, as they usually outlast clay litters, the difference in cost may be minimal—even insignificant—when you consider their environmental and user friendliness.

One of the newer members of the cat litter team is crystals. The crystals were very popular when first introduced, but they seem to have peaked in popularity. Still, they're an excellent option for many cat owners. Made from sodium silicate, they are very porous and absorb more urine and urine odor than any of the other products so far introduced. A single bag can last one cat approximately one month. You simply scoop the feces and occasionally stir the crystals to ensure they contact any urine at the bottom of the pan. When most of the crystals have begun to yellow, it's time to replace them. Some brands offer low-tracking formulas. However, if you do step on one, you'll know it instantly, as they're large enough for a minor "ouch" if you forget to wear your slippers.

There are other litter products out there, with new ones arriving on the scene regularly. Don't assume that the old litter you've been using for decades is your only option.

For some reason, many cat owners seem hesitant to try out new litters. (Can it be that the cat's conservative nature is shared by cat owners?) Considering the potential benefit associated with the newer products,

I think it's worth the small risk involved to give them a try. It's true that cats don't like change without their consent. (If they do consent to something, get it in writing.) Sometimes they may be offended by a new litter's odor; other times they'll be put off by a texture change. So if you're brave enough to try a new litter, introduce it gradually. Mix a small amount of the new litter into the old litter. The next time you change the litter, increase the amount of new litter in the mixture. Keep increasing the ratio of new to old each time you replace the litter. Be patient! Once the new litter's ratio reaches about two-thirds of the total, it's probably safe to eliminate the old litter completely.

CHAPTER 13

Your Pet's Pets

There are many intelligent species in the universe. They are all owned by cats.

—Anonymous

Forgive me for frivolously implying there's anything pet-ish about parasites; they're nobody's pets. Most of my customers fail to realize there's a link between nutrition and many of the parasites plaguing our pet population. A healthy, well-nourished pet can deal with a few parasites without suffering any serious effects. It's when health conditions allow parasites to gain the upper hand that trouble begins. Some parasites gravitate toward animals that are vulnerable; the very young, elderly, weak, or ill pet with a compromised immune system is a preferred target. Surface and intestinal parasites, such as fleas and hookworms, can turn a mildly ill pet into a very ill pet if left unchecked. Intestinal parasites such as whipworm compete with the host for nutrients in the digestive tract, robbing your pet of valuable nourishment while enjoying their freeloading lifestyle and potentially creating chronic digestive problems in the process. Others, like hookworm, feast off blood, debilitating your pet when their numbers increase.

If intestinal parasites are left untreated, your pet can eventually become dehydrated from resultant diarrhea, malnourished from inadequate nutrition, anemic from blood loss, and suffer excessive weight loss. Additionally, both internal and external parasites can cause allergic and autoimmune reactions that will further impair the health of Whiskers or Spot. A cat or dog enjoying a nutritious diet will be more resistant to parasites and their impact and recover faster follow-ing treatment. It's also worth noting that a nutrition-poor pet diet may be a nutrition-rich parasite diet. Foods reported to stimulate intestinal parasite growth includes gluten from grains such as corn and wheat, along with sugar and artificial sweeteners; yet another reason to avoid grain-rich diets and anything with sugar. It's also worth repeating here that raw diets with improperly sourced or prepared ingredients may contain intestinal parasites.

To provide detailed information on every parasite dwelling in our cat and dog populations would entail writing another book. Instead, I'll limit the information here to those few parasites that I most frequently come across in dealing with my customers. When I lived in the country we used to jokingly claim there's no such thing as one mouse in the house. Well, there's no such thing as one flea on your pet . . . and that's no joke.

FLEAS

In addition to being a nuisance in themselves, fleas can cause allergic reactions from their saliva and, when ingested by your pet, become a major source of tapeworm. In warm climates, fleas are a constant prob-lem. In colder regions, where I live, they're a seasonal irritation. How-ever, once fleas get into your home the season can become very long; I've had customers complain about fleas when the snow was falling. Dealing with a flea infestation can turn your home into a battleground; it has always been a wonder to me that so many pet owners wait until a problem develops before taking action. Personally, I have always found that an ounce of prevention is the best, easiest, least expensive, and simplest solution where fleas are concerned. The bottom line is that you should implement flea control before you have a flea problem.

There are over two thousand flea species, but the main pest we com-monly deal with in North America is the cat flea; ironic, as the cat flea isn't feline specific when seeking a good place to reside. Anything warm, furry, and able to provide a blood meal will do. Today there are a large variety of products available that are inexpensive, easy to use, and effective in controlling fleas. These products fall into two groups designed to either combat a problem or prevent a problem. Prior to spending your money, you need to determine which problem you're dealing with. If you're preventing a problem, you're one giant step ahead of the fleas.

Flea Prevention

Flea/tick collars, spot-on drops, and oral chew tablets provide convenient protection for your pets and are easy to apply. They are also affordable. Those you obtain from a pet supply store are effective and are usually less expensive than that provided by veterinarians. Some flea/tick collars need to be activated, usually with a quick stretch before being placed on the pet, so read the package instructions before using. The instructions will also tell you the collar's effective life, usually from three to nine months. Because of the toxicity associated with flea collars, I don't recommend them if pregnant women or small children will come into direct contact with the collar or pet. Collars, while still popular, are slowly giving way to drops and oral tablets.

Drops (spot-on treatment) are usually applied between the back of the neck and shoulders on small or medium-sized pets. For larger pets, it is often recommended to apply half the drops to the shoulder area and the remainder to the rump, just above the tail. Drops normally protect one pet for one month and are usually weight related (under thirty pounds, over thirty pounds). Like collars, they may not be the best product if small children are in the home. Drops are considered to be more effective than collars.

Note: Wash your hands thoroughly after applying a collar or drops.

Oral flea control products are becoming increasingly popular, both for convenience and safety. They are available in a flavored, chewable form for both cats and dogs, or a liquid in some cases. They are the safest flea treatment where small children, pregnant women, and other pets are concerned, as the chemicals will not be present on the pet's skin or hair. Like drops, they are considered to be very effective. Oral products targeting live fleas have a very fast kill effect. You will likely also require a companion oral product targeting flea eggs and larvae with an insect growth regulator (IGR). This ingredient works to sterilize flea eggs and prevent larvae from developing.

While an IGR is often included in collars and drops to provide a one-two punch by killing adult fleas and their offspring, oral products are either a live flea killer or an IGR (you'll require both: I anticipate a rapid rise in popularity for oral flea prevention when pharmaceutical companies figure out how to combine both the kill and IGR ingredients into a single dose). The inclusion of an IGR ingredient is important. I've had innumerable complaints over the years from customers advising their flea products failed to work. They worked fine. The problem results when new batches of fleas hatch from unsterilized eggs randomly dropped around the house. These new fleas, hatching at various times, will quickly find their way to your pet, leaving you with the erroneous impression the fleas were never killed off in the first place. Each new batch of fleas sends you back to square one. An IGR will prevent this from happening by disrupting the flea life cycle.

Some flea control products can only be obtained from a veterinarian or with a vet prescription. Most will kill both fleas and ticks, and some will also control a range of intestinal parasites and mites. I can foresee the day when a single product will control all parasites—surface pests such as fleas, ticks, and mites, and intestinal parasites such as heartworm and tapeworm.

Warnings: If you live in a dog and cat home, some flea products for Spot may be unsafe for Whiskers if the two come into physical contact. For example, permethrin, while effective as a flea control for dogs, can be fatal to a cat. (If concerned, read the package information or contact the company before purchasing.)

Do not implement combinations of flea/tick treatments. By that I mean don't use drops AND a collar, or a collar AND an oral treatment. All of these products are effective on their own. In addition to wasting your money through redundant applications, you may be endangering your pet's health with a potentially harmful combination of chemicals. (I provide this warning as I have customers who, in their haste to eliminate fleas, have doubled up when applying flea control products.)

Flea Control

What if you have skipped prevention and are now facing a flea problem in your home? A single adult female flea can lay up to fifty eggs a day, so this problem can escalate quickly. While the eggs are deposited on your pet's hair, they usually fall off, eventually hatching from wherever they land. If fleas are still restricted to your cat or dog (nobody else is being bitten), then a flea shampoo followed by applying a flea collar, drops, or oral tablets, and a few days of rigorously vacuuming the house, will likely solve your problem.

If you're unlucky in that the problem has evolved to a point where the two-foots in the home are experiencing flea bites, you have an infestation and need to take fast action to get on top of the situation. Consider a flea premise spray as an initial step. These aerosol insecticide sprays are available at pet supply stores and, unlike regular household insecticides, will usually contain an IGR ingredient to sterilize flea eggs. Further, the treatment should provide a residual action that will continue to work for some time. You will need sufficient spray to treat all rooms in the home, even rooms where pets aren't allowed as, given enough time, fleas will find their way into every nook and cranny in your home. If it's an extremely bad situation, with fleas everywhere, you might also consider hiring a pest control company to fog your home.

Once you've sprayed the home, it's time for a flea bath, as that's the fastest way to rid your pet of the fleas roaming over its body. A flea shampoo is a quick fix, though, providing no residual kill action, and it should be followed up with long-acting products such as a collar, drops, or oral control. In order to make the bath as effective as possible, there are some important steps to follow.

Tip: Before you start Step 1, put on a short-sleeve shirt like a T-shirt . . . or no shirt. You want bare arms to quickly detect any escaping fleas jumping from the pet to you. Fleas can jump about twelve inches (thirty centimeters), so keep your pet at arm's reach as best you can.

Step 1: Place your pet in a tub or large sink of lukewarm water. Starting from the front, slowly and thoroughly soak all of the head and face with water, including between the ears and under the jaw and throat area. Once the head area is completely soaked with water, wait for a couple of minutes before proceeding. Fleas hate water; any fleas in the head area will move rearward seeking a dry location. Continue soaking the dog/cat, wetting it down thoroughly and slooooooooowly, from front to rear, soaking the chest and belly areas also. Your objective is to herd as many fleas as possible toward the pet's rear end. Once you've reached the rear, soak that area thoroughly, including under and along the tail. At this point the fleas will be feeling a bit desperate.

Step 2: Starting again from front to back, apply a generous amount of the flea shampoo to your pet and work it up into a good lather all over the body except the head. Avoid getting any shampoo in your pet's eyes or ears. I only apply a small amount of shampoo between the ears, along with a more generous application under the jaw and down the neck. Be thorough in applying shampoo around and under the base of the tail, as it's a favorite flea hideout.

Step 3: Wait! Most flea shampoos require a waiting period of three to five minutes, the longer the better. This period maximizes the shampoo's kill effect on fleas.

Step 4: Thoroughly rinse your pet with clean, lukewarm water. Again, start at the head and work rearward. You want the entire shampoo residue rinsed off.

Step 5: If you are dealing with a lot of fleas on your pet, you might consider repeating steps 2, 3, and 4. A second application will assuredly eliminate any live fleas that escaped the initial treatment. If not repeating, go to step 6.

Step 6: Subject to the size of the pet being treated, have sufficient towels handy to remove excess water from all body areas. After toweling, she/he will still be a bit damp. I recommend keeping your pet in the home until it is completely dry, especially if it is cool outside.

Step 7: Once dry (no dampness), apply a flea/tick collar, drops, or oral tablets.

Most dogs will cooperate, even begrudgingly, with a bath. Some cats will assume you have murder on your mind and react to a bath accordingly. With sharp teeth and four sets of nasty claws, bathing an angry, uncooperative feline can prove to be a futile, even dangerous exercise. When faced with a fiercely uncooperative cat, skip the bath. Apply flea drops, oral chews, or a good flea collar. Results won't materialize as quickly as with a bath, but within a few hours the resident flea population will go into decline.

For safety's sake, we're going to assume that some of the fleas have escaped the flea spray you initially used. These escapees will likely consist of adult and juvenile fleas and unhatched flea eggs. First, run any washable pet bedding (including your bedding if the pet sleeps on your bed) through a washing machine cycle, as that will kill any live fleas, larvae, and eggs. Next, become the neighborhood vacuuming champion. Vacuum furniture, floors, rugs, and anywhere your pet has walked or lain, and do this chore on a daily basis until the infestation has been defeated.

Tip: To prevent fleas escaping from a vacuum, vacuum up two or three mothballs before going after the fleas; the mothballs will kill fleas and eggs captured by the vacuum.

TICKS

Fleas create infestations both on the pet and in the home, and ticks, fortunately, don't do this. While fleas are a significant source of tapeworms, unlike ticks, they aren't normally associated with serious diseases. Ticks, while not as profuse as fleas when on our pets, are often the more dangerous as they can be carriers of Lyme disease, Colorado fever, and a host of other diseases. Ticks are related to spiders. They prefer a warm, humid environment and, like fleas, require blood meals for survival.

There is a great deal of information available on the Internet regarding the removal of ticks from Spot or Whiskers. Much of the information is valid, but some is misleading or outright erroneous. If you live in a tick-infested area, check your pet daily for ticks. In other areas, it's wise to check your dog if it's been for a walk in a potential tick area, or your cat if it has been allowed to wander. Here's my contribution to tick removal: forget all of the Internet advice and buy a tick key from a pet supply store. These simple gadgets are inexpensive, easy to use, and very effective. Be sure to clean and disinfect the wound after removal, and do the same with the tick key after each use—and thoroughly wash your hands after removing a tick (in fact, it's a good idea to wear light kitchen gloves when dealing with ticks). The Centers for Disease Control recommends avoiding popular folklore remedies such as "painting" the tick with nail polish or petroleum jelly, or using heat to make the tick detach from the skin.

Most of the products mentioned in the discussion on fleas will also control ticks, so I won't repeat them here.

Warning: Many flea and tick products are not suitable for use on kittens or puppies under eight weeks old, others under four weeks, and may not be safe for pregnant/nursing mothers. Read the package information before applying any parasite controls to these pets, or consult with your veterinarian.

THE TERRIBLE TAPEWORM

Following fleas and ticks, the most common parasite my customers encounter is tapeworm. These yucky pests infect both cats and dogs. If we are not careful, they can pass to humans, although it is uncommon for adult humans to contract tapeworm. Young children are more at risk when playing in areas contaminated with tapeworm eggs, such as sandboxes used as a litter box by a passing cat.

Tapeworms inhabit your pet's small intestine. Lacking a mouth, they absorb nutrients directly through their skin as food passes along the intestine, thus robbing vital nutrition from your pet. There are several species commonly found in cats and dogs and, in general, tapeworm infestation is worldwide. Adult worms can grow up to twenty inches. What you see issuing from your pet's anus are mature, egg-laden segments that have been cast off from the back end of the worm. When these pods dry out, they rupture, releasing their store of eggs. Eggs can be ingested by a louse or a flea larva and develop into an immature form while residing in these intermediate hosts. When Spot or Whiskers ingests the flea host while grooming themselves, the worm commences developing into its mature form. Cats ingesting mice are also at risk of getting tapeworm.

The initial diagnosis that your pet has tapeworms usually comes from observing your pet's feces immediately after a bowel movement, as segments will often be passed along with the stool. You might also spot them around your pet's anus or on bedding. Tapeworm segments are about the size of a grain of rice, but they are flatter and, unlike a grain of rice, they can move when fresh. Their color is normally white and may have a pink or yellow undertone.

There is no foolproof method of defending your pet against a tapeworm. That being said, when you consider that most tapeworm problems result from ingesting fleas, the application of flea controls goes a long way toward preventing a potential tapeworm problem. If those measures have failed and you identify tapeworm segments issuing from your pet's anus, treatment should be implemented immediately. Appropriate medication can be obtained from a pet supply store or veterinarian. Both sources of supply provide effective products, but it may be less expensive from a pet supply store. Treatment normally consists of a series of tablets orally administered to Whiskers or Spot over a period of days. As some pets will reject tablets, it's okay to crush them and mix it with something to mask the medicine, such as canned food, ketchup, or yogurt. There is also a great product, Pill Pockets (greenies. com), sold in cat or dog versions and available from pet supply stores, which will assist in getting that important pill into your four-footer.

Note: Until the tapeworm situation has been brought under control, keep small children away from the pet, its bedding, and other areas the pet frequents in the home. Wash hands thoroughly after any contact with tapeworm segments, or after picking up dog poop and cleaning cat litter boxes.

THE HEARTACHE OF HEARTWORM

No discussion of pet parasites can be complete without covering heartworm. It's a popular topic: Google *heartworm in dogs* and you'll get about 4,600,000 results and nearly the same number for cats. Heartworm is common throughout most of the United States and southern Canada, where warmer temperatures favor the parasite's development in mosquito hosts; the disease appears to be spreading as climate change provides higher temperatures and longer seasons supporting increased mosquito activity. Any pet likely to come into frequent contact with mosquitoes should be on heartworm prevention medication. Most mammals can be infected with heartworm, including humans (very rare), but canines seem to suffer more than others, although there is increasing concern regarding the degree of incidence in our feline population. Along with mosquitoes, mammals are required for a series of developmental stages in the life of a heartworm. When a mosquito bites your pet, heartworm microfilariae can pass from the insect into the wound and in time develop into mature heartworms in your pet's body. When these worms eventually breed, their microfilariae are passed back to mosquitoes when the pet is bitten on a future occasion. In this way, the long and very complicated heartworm life cycle manages to repeat itself. It's just one more reason to hate mosquitoes; no mosquitoes, no heartworm!

While even an indoor cat, or a dog that gets walked once daily on a city street in broad daylight for thirty minutes, can become infected, those pets are at low risk. Even if it does meet up with a mosquito, not all mosquitoes are carriers. That being said, heartworm is a dangerous disease with a double edge; left unchecked, it can prove fatal. Ridding a pet of heartworm is a very dangerous process that can also prove fatal if not managed properly. For this reason, eliminating heartworms should only be attempted under veterinarian supervision. Unless you live in a climate not favorable to heartworm, both your cat and dog should be on heartworm prevention medication.

Warning: Mosquitoes aren't the only insect benefiting from warmer weather. Fleas and ticks are also enjoying global warming trends; in cooler climates their threat now commences earlier and lasts longer. If you used to commence flea prevention in mid-May, consider starting as early as the first of April.

ROUNDWORM, HOOKWORM, WHIPWORM

And you thought we were finished discussing worms! These parasites represent three good reasons why Whiskers and Spot should be dewormed on a regular basis. Unlike tapeworm, their presence is more difficult to detect. If suspicious, the only sure way to identify the problem is through a fecal flotation test for worm eggs performed by your vet. Symptoms warranting your suspicion will include rapid weight loss, excessive diarrhea, bloody diarrhea, pot belly, weakness, lethargy, or anemia.

Some of these internal parasites will rob your pet of nutrients by ingesting digested food; others will feed from the blood supply drawn from the intestinal wall. Eradicating these parasites should be done under veterinary supervision as stages of treatment are usually required and the timing of each stage can be crucial to success. Killing adult worms is often the easy part, but dead adult worms are not dead larvae, and the offspring also must be attacked at specific times. Left unchecked, the actions of some of these parasites can prove fatal to your pet.

EAR MITES

These little monsters are a common problem, especially in puppies and kittens. Like ticks, mites are related to spiders. Ear mites spread quickly; just a brief contact with another infected animal will allow them to move to a new host. They seem to like cats more than dogs and can also be a problem for ferrets and rabbits. As they are so tiny, it's unlikely you'll be able to spot them unless you possess some of Superman's wondrous vision. However, the telltale signs they leave behind provide all the clues you require as to their presence. Your first clue will come from noticing excessive scratching in the vicinity of the ears and head shaking. If you peer inside the ear, you may see a crumbly, brownish-blackish substance on the skin down toward the canal. Using a damp cotton swab, swipe the inside of the ear where the substance appears. (Never insert a swab too far into the ear.) If the residue staining the swab is reddish, it's from blood and confirms the presence of ear mites. Sometimes a yeasty odor will be detectable, but this can be confusing, leading to the assumption that you're dealing with a yeast infection rather than a mite infestation.

Products to rid your pet of ear mites are available from pet supply retailers and veterinarians. They're easy to use and effective. In serious cases, you may wish to use a veterinarian service, especially if the mites have created excessive debris in the ear or if your pet experiences an ongoing ear infection. Some flea control products will also eliminate mites.

MANGE MITES

Sarcoptic mange, sometimes known as scabies, is the most common form of mange. In the Introduction, you met Frisky the Undocked Poodle. When we were still living in the country, Frisky contracted sarcoptic mange. At that time, this mange was a relatively rare event in our area, probably arriving with the recent migration of coyotes into the district. It was sufficiently uncommon as to warrant two or three visits to our vet before the problem was properly diagnosed. Frisky certainly needed the vet's aid because he was chewing his back end off—literally. His rear looked like raw meat and there wasn't one second in a day when he wasn't suffering.

Back then, the only treatment for sarcoptic mange involved dipping the dog in a treated bath (like a sheep dip) to kill the mites. One treatment of this, the vet advised, will clean up the problem for good. She was wrong about that; the second treatment finally did the trick. Today, while the dip is still used, the veterinarian community has superior weapons in its arsenal. The new treatments are easily administered orally or as drops, are very effective, and provide fast results.

These mites can infect humans and cats, but they really don't like us or cats as hosts, so the infestation usually doesn't continue. However, cats can contract notoedric mange, a close cousin to the sarcoptic pest. The symptoms usually appear as itching and scabbing on a cat's facial area. Treatment for notoedric mange is the same as for the sarcoptic variety.

There is also a demodectic mange mite, sometimes referred to as red mange. Unlike other mites, they aren't considered to be contagious. These mites are so common that almost all dogs have them; however, it's rare for this type of mange to become a problem. If a problem develops, it's usually a result of the dog's immune system being compromised by other conditions, which may include a lack of good nutrition from a poor diet. When this happens, these insignificant mites can take advantage of the deteriorated situation and become detrimental to your pet by turning a benign situation into a serious health problem.

CHAPTER 14

All Good Things Come to an End

A pet is never truly forgotten until it is no longer remembered.

—Lacie Petitto

While somewhat off topic in a book focused primarily on nutrition-related matters, dealing with a loved pet's death is a subject that has too frequently come up with my customers. I said *somewhat off topic*, as good nutrition even comes into play here. A cat or dog eating a nutritious, healthy diet stands a better chance of greater longevity, as well as enjoying a better quality of life in its senior years, a pleasant benefit for both pet and paropet.

Often, when a pet passes away, my customer will come into the store and advise me of the event as, in many cases, I have shared a small part in their pet's life. At those times, I'm like a bartender dealing with someone whose marriage has just broken up; it just isn't good. I keep a handy box of tissues beneath the counter for them . . . and sometimes for me. I like to think it helps them a little to discuss the circumstances of their bereavement. Having been in the same position myself on more than one occasion, I certainly have empathy for their loss.

I love Ms. Petitto's above quote, but when is a loved pet no longer remembered? I remember all of my dogs and cats. Sure, I don't actively think of them every day, but now and then something will happen, forcing me or another family member to recall a happy incident involving Busted, or Frisky, or Cinnamon, or Blondie, or any of the other wonderful companions who have shared our lives as a cherished part of the family. I remember them all, and I wish I could have each of them back with me.

One of the most difficult decisions we pet parents have to make in our lives involves having to put a loved cat or dog to sleep. It is an extremely difficult step, often involving a lot of soul-searching even when we know, deep in our hearts, that it's the right thing to do—not the right thing for us; rather, it's the right thing for our loved ones.

When your pet passes away, it's like a black hole suddenly enters your home and sucks out some of the life and vitality that once occupied each room, leaving a vacancy that, until then, you never imagined could exist. When it happens, you realize a life is much more than just a warm body. A life can maintain a presence, even when absent.

Frequently, the customer will, in their grief, vow never to go through the pain of separation again. No more pets. Ever! I just nod in agreement. Right! Never again! What I do understand right then—and they don't—is that the vacancy in the home stubbornly refuses to vanish. It's like a mooching relative who's moved into your basement bedroom for a month and is still there three years later. It won't go away. Sure enough, two, or four, or six months later, they pop into the store with a big smile to inform me about their new family member. They are excited and happy. And they are always astounded at how different the new adoptee's personality is from that of their deceased pet. It is truly amazing how a cat or dog manages to seamlessly insert itself into our hearts, and it doesn't take them very long to access our hearts, a time span often measured in only a few heartbeats.

We don't even realize that the vacancy has quietly vanished, now a fond memory. That's the incredible power of a new life.

The problem with our cats and dogs is that, compared with humans, they have such short lives. This means we will always be faced with dealing with their deaths. We never think of this when we welcome them into our hearts. The realization becomes obvious when, only a few years later, we are faced with the unpleasant reality of their passing. Why do we inflict this pain on ourselves? Why, after suffering the loss of a pet, do we often adopt another cat or dog weeks or months later? Are we insane?

I don't think we're insane. I believe we intuitively understand that the unconditional love we receive from our pets in those few short years is a treasured gift far greater in value than our grief at their passing.

THE FACTS OF THE MATTER

I have long admired the selfless endeavors of the thousands of staff and volunteers who devote time and energy in assisting the hapless animals that find themselves in rescue shelters. These dedicated folks raise funds to pay veterinarian bills for spay/neuter programs, injuries, vaccinations, and more. They investigate and rescue animals from environments that are demeaning, violent, and cruel. They work to rehabilitate our animals, heal them, and find good homes for them. They are angels. They deserve our support. Here are a few reasons why:

The Top Ten Reasons for Pet Relinquishment to Shelters in the United States (petpopulation.org):

Dogs	Cats
1. Moving	1. Too many in house
2. Landlord issues	2. Allergies
3. Cost of pet maintenance	3. Moving
4. No time for pet	4. Cost of pet maintenance
5. Inadequate facilities	5. Landlord issues
6. Too many pets in home	6. No homes for littermates
7. Pet illness	7. House soiling
8. Personal problems	8. Personal problems
9. Biting	9. Inadequate facilities
10. No homes for littermates	10. Doesn't get along with other pets

Facts about U.S. Animal Shelters (aspca.org):

There are about five thousand community animal shelters nationwide that are independent; there is no national organization monitoring these shelters. The terms *humane society* and *SPCA* are generic; shelters using those names are not part of the ASPCA or the Humane Society of the United States. Currently, no government institution or animal organization is responsible for tabulating national statistics for the animal protection movement.

- Approximately five million to seven million companion animals enter animal shelters nationwide every year, and approximately three million to four million are euthanized (60 percent of dogs and 70 percent of cats). Shelter intakes are about evenly divided between those animals relinquished by owners and those picked up by animal control. These are national estimates; the percentage of euthanasia may vary from state to state.

- According to the National Council on Pet Population Study and Policy (NCPPSP), less than 2 percent of cats and only 15 to 20 percent of dogs are returned to their owners. Most of these were identified with tags, tattoos, or microchips.
- Some 25 percent of dogs who enter local shelters are purebred. (Source: NCPPSP)
- Only 10 percent of the animals received by shelters have been spayed or neutered, while 78 percent of pet dogs and 88 percent of pet cats are spayed or neutered, according to the American Pet Products Association. (Source: APPA)
- More than 20 percent of people who leave dogs in shelters adopted them from a shelter. (Source: NCPPSP)

Facts about Pet Ownership in the United States (aspc.org):

- About 62 percent of all households in the United States have a pet. (Source: APPA)
- About 78.2 million dogs and about 86.4 million cats are owned in the United States. (Source: APPA)
- According to NCPPSP, about 65 percent of pet owners acquire their pets free or at low cost.
- The majority of pets are obtained from acquaintances and family members. Some 26 percent of dogs are purchased from breeders, 20 to 30 percent of cats and dogs are adopted from shelters and rescues, and 2 to 10 percent are purchased from pet shops.
- At least one-third of cats are acquired as strays. (Source: APPA)
- More than 20 percent of people who leave dogs in shelters adopted them from a shelter. (Source: NCPPSP)
- The cost of spaying and neutering a pet is less than the cost of raising puppies or kittens for one year.
- The average cost of basic food, supplies, medical care, and training for a dog or cat is $600 to $900 annually. Some 78 percent of pet dogs and 88 percent of pet cats are spayed or neutered. (Source: APPA)

Facts about Pet Overpopulation in the United States (aspc.org):

- It is impossible to determine how many stray dogs and cats live in the United States; estimates for cats alone range up to seventy million.

- The average number of litters a fertile cat produces is one to two a year; the average number of kittens is four to six per litter.
- The average number of litters a fertile dog produces is one a year; the average number of puppies is four to six.
- Owned cats and dogs generally live longer, healthier lives than strays.
- Many strays are lost pets that were not kept properly indoors or provided with identification.
- Only 10 percent of the animals received by shelters have been spayed or neutered, while 78 percent of pet dogs and 88 percent of pet cats are spayed or neutered.
- The cost of spaying or neutering a pet is less than the cost of raising puppies or kittens for a year.

In 2006, nearly half of pet owners, or 49.7 percent, considered their pets to be family members (avma.org).
Percent of households owning dogs / 37.2 percent; cats / 32.4 percent
Number of households owning dogs / 43,021,000; cats / 37,460,000
Average number pets/household dogs / 1.7; cats / 2.2

Pet Overpopulation Statistics United States (humanesociety.org):
Estimated number of cats and dogs entering shelters each year: six to eight million
Estimated number of cats and dogs euthanized by shelters each year: three to four million
Estimated number of cats and dogs adopted from shelters each year: three to four million
Estimated number of cats and dogs reclaimed by owners from shelters each year: 30 percent of dogs and 2 to 5 percent of cats

A portion of the author's royalties will be donated to animal rescue organizations in the United States and Canada.

Index

About the Author

David G. Wellock has owned and operated a Global Pet Foods retail store for thirteen years. During this period he acquired a unique knowledge of topics from pet food manufacturers to pets—and everything in between. David led the charge in his community by introducing the new, healthy pet diets that appeared in the marketplace over a decade ago. Educating pet parents became a part of his program, a personal mission culminating with this book.

David has twice served as a member of the Global Pet Foods Franchisee Advisory Board. He worked in the duty-free industry for many years and is a former director of the Frontier Duty Free Association, an American/Canadian organization.